INTERMITTENT
FASTING
MADE EASY

Use Intermittent Fasting to Lose Fat, Build Muscle,
Boost Energy, and Get the Most Out of Life

THOMAS DeLAUER

FAIR WINDS

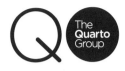

Inspiring | Educating | Creating | Entertaining

Brimming with creative inspiration, how-to projects, and useful information to enrich your everyday life, Quarto.com is a favorite destination for those pursuing their interests and passions.

First Published in 2022 by Fair Winds Press, an imprint of The Quarto Group, 100 Cummings Center, Suite 265-D, Beverly, MA 01915, USA.
T (978) 282-9590 F (978) 283-2742 QuartoKnows.com

Fair Winds Press titles are also available at discount for retail, wholesale, promotional, and bulk purchase. For details, contact the Special Sales Manager by email at specialsales@quarto.com or by mail at The Quarto Group, Attn: Special Sales Manager, 100 Cummings Center, Suite 265-D, Beverly, MA 01915, USA.

26 25 24 23 22   1 2 3 4 5

ISBN: 978-0-7603-7386-6

Digital edition published in 2022
eISBN: 978-0-7603-7387-3

Library of Congress Cataloging-in-Publication Data

Names: DeLauer, Thomas, author.
Title: Intermittent fasting made easy : next-level hacks to supercharge fat loss, boost energy, and build muscle / Thomas DeLauer.
Description: Beverly : Fair Winds Press, 2022. | Includes bibliographical references and index. | Summary: "Intermittent Fasting Made Easy is the ordinary person's best practice guide to doing intermittent fasting optimally, effectively, and safely, written by top nutrition and fitness expert and YouTube sensation Thomas DeLauer"-- Provided by publisher.
Identifiers: LCCN 2021043423 (print) | LCCN 2021043424 (ebook) | ISBN 9780760373866 (trade paperback) | ISBN 9780760373873 (ebook)
Subjects: LCSH: Intermittent fasting. | Reducing diets.
Classification: LCC RM222.2 .D457 2022 (print) | LCC RM222.2 (ebook) | DDC 613.2/5--dc23/eng/20211007
LC record available at https://lccn.loc.gov/2021043423
LC ebook record available at https://lccn.loc.gov/2021043424

Design and page layout: Laura Shaw Design
Cover Image: Glenn Scott Photography and J. R. Carino (portrait)
Illustration: adapted from Shutterstock

Printed in China

ALSO BY THOMAS DeLAUER

The New Mediterranean Diet Cookbook: The Optimal Keto-Friendly Diet that Burns Fat, Promotes Longevity, and Prevents Chronic Disease (with Martina Slajerova, Dr. Nicholas Norwitz, and Rohan Kashid)

To my mother, who always instilled in me to march to the beat of a different drum and to never take "no" for an answer if it's something you're passionate about.

And to my wife, Amber, who has stood by my side since we were teenagers, consistently "zagging" when everyone else was "zigging."

CONTENTS

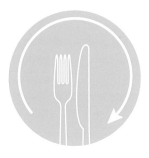

INTRODUCTION

Do It for Yourself

TEN YEARS AGO, I weighed 280 pounds (127 kg). Looking at me now, you may find that hard to believe, but it's true, and I have the pictures and stretch marks to prove it. I was 100 pounds (45.3 kg) overweight and the poster child for unhealthy. I was borderline diabetic, had acid reflux, and was hypertensive. Worst of all, I felt like total garbage as I battled severe depression and anxiety. I am not just some in-shape guy who has always been fit. I know what it's like to be overweight and to struggle to lose weight. I know what it's like to try to make a change.

Growing up, I was an active kid and young adult, participating in sports such as cross-country, track, and rugby. I was in pretty good shape when I left school. That didn't last long. Once I started working, my priorities became providing for my family, chasing coin,

and success. Being a health care recruiter, and then an executive with an ancillary lab services company that provided testing solutions to physicians and medical groups, was rewarding but very demanding. Tight deadlines, early mornings, late nights, and after-hours wining and dining of potential clients stressed me out. So, I ate . . . and ate . . . and ate—and I didn't move much more than it took to walk from my front door to the car to my office and back again. You can see where this is going. The funny thing is, I didn't even realize how much weight I was gaining because I'd gotten so far out of touch with my body. I had tunnel vision, and all I could see was my career.

But, as the health scares piled on and my relationship with my wife, Amber, suffered, there was no getting around it: Something needed to change.

The top-notch doctors and experts in the health care community whom I worked with and managed became my teachers and, alongside Amber, my support system. From them, I learned so much about what goes into making someone healthy. When some of the physicians I most respected suggested intermittent fasting, I was all in—mainly because the idea sounded simple and easy. All I had to do was keep my eating to within an eight-hour window. That, I could handle. With intermittent fasting, I dropped more than 100 pounds (45.3 kg) in a little over one year. My health stabilized, my mood improved, and my marriage got back on track. Intermittent fasting became a way of life and now, more than a decade later, I credit it with helping me keep the weight off, maximizing my health, and helping me find my passion and purpose.

You see, while I was undergoing this physical transformation, my mental and emotional outlook changed as well: I realized that the intense pressure of corporate life and chasing money wasn't the life I wanted. I wanted to have a family and actually be present in their lives. I also wanted to help people in the same way I had been helped. Discovering why my body composition changed with intermittent fasting and why my body responded differently to various foods ignited an interest in biochemistry and how the body works. The more I dove into the research on intermittent fasting and nutrition, the more excited I became—and the more I was convinced that if others knew about it, they'd be excited too.

My YouTube channel was born out of a desire to explain the latest research and information about intermittent fasting and the way the human body functions. I'm not a doctor and I don't pretend to be one. But I am good at communicating complex subject matter in an accessible, down-to-earth way, and I always back up everything with science and evidence. I consider myself a knowledgeable expert, and that knowledge propels me forward on my health journey. Over the years, my channel has grown to nearly 2.7 million subscribers with more than fifteen million views per month and I've helped thousands of people reach their health goals. Along the way, I've seen what an extraordinary motivator knowledge is, empowering people to make positive changes and successfully incorporate intermittent fasting into their lifestyle. It makes sense. When you understand what's happening in your body and why certain actions lead to more beneficial outcomes, you're more likely to pursue your goals and stick with them. My motto remains: Pursue results, reinforce with science.

That's where this book comes in, offering everything you need to know about the science of intermittent fasting along with an easy-to-follow action plan to help you get going and get the most out of the process. I worked with the best in the health space and everything I share—the tips, strategies, and advice—I share because I know it works and will help you become the best possible version of yourself.

INTERMITTENT FASTING IS FOR YOU

Let's get this out of the way right now: Intermittent fasting is not a trend or a fad. Putting aside the fact that people have been fasting throughout history, intermittent fasting is a healthy, science-backed approach to losing weight and upgrading your overall physical and mental performance. It's also a pretty simple formula: Not eating for a set period of time kicks your body into a fasting state that brings with it an incredible array of benefits. Instead of eating throughout the day, you concentrate your daily meals into one window of time, flipping a metabolic switch in your body that promotes fat burning, gut health, insulin sensitivity, and mental sharpness, among a host of other pluses.[1]

Whether you are looking to get into amazing shape or simply to feel your absolute best, you are in the right place to find out how to:

- Bust a weight loss plateau
- Torch body fat while preserving muscle[2]
- Reverse insulin resistance[3]
- Reduce inflammation[4]
- Improve gut health and restore your microbiome[5]
- Give your brain a boost and increase your attention, focus, and memory[6]
- Have more energy[7]
- Live longer[8]

The impressive health advantages you receive from intermittent fasting are reason enough to make it part of your lifestyle, but if you're on the fence or thinking it's only for a certain type of person, think again. Consider:

→ **It's for everybody.** Okay, there are certain people who should not do intermittent fasting (see page 21), but by and large, no matter where you are on your health journey, you will benefit from intermittent fasting. And, if you're a busy, high-performing individual or have a physically or mentally taxing job (parents and shift workers, I'm looking at you), you stand to gain significantly by upping your energy and brain power. Intermittent fasting also helps regulate sleep patterns, a phenomenal bonus, especially if you travel a lot.[9]

→ **It's flexible.** You can allocate your fasting period to whenever you like and for however long you like based on what works for you. There's no rigid schedule or timetable that you need to follow.

→ **It makes life easier.** The biggest challenges to healthy living are time and convenience. Intermittent fasting has both of these issues covered. No one has a lot of time. Everything moves at warp speed. It's a lot easier not to eat than to try to figure out what you should eat or what "eating healthy" means. It also takes a lot less time not to eat than it does to eat unhealthy foods. I don't care how convenient it is to zip through a fast food drive-through window. Nothing is more convenient than not idling there in the first place. Let's be real: Meal prep can be a hassle. With intermittent fasting, you can nix a lot of that weekly assembly line of organizing chicken breasts and broccoli in a row of glassware containers.

→ **It fits all types of eating plans:** keto, paleo, vegan, vegetarian, you name it. Intermittent fasting affords tremendous flexibility with your diet. I advocate for eating clean (we'll cover that in chapter 6), but it's up to you how you eat outside your fasting window.

→ **It doesn't require expensive specialty foods.** The start-up costs for intermittent fasting are nil, and you may even save money because you'll be skipping some meals.

→ **It can help you become the best version of you, from the inside out.** You'll harness your inner drive and discipline and strengthen your mental game, which will help you unlock your full potential in every arena.

I know exactly where you are because I've been there, too—wondering if all this sounds too good to be true, and even if it isn't, uncertain you'll be able to make intermittent fasting stick. I won't sugarcoat it. Research backs up all the benefits I highlight but everybody— and body—is different. Your results will be unique to you. What I can promise is that with *Intermittent Fasting Made Easy*, you'll know why intermittent fasting works, what to do every step of the way, and how to take care of the most common challenges associated with the practice.

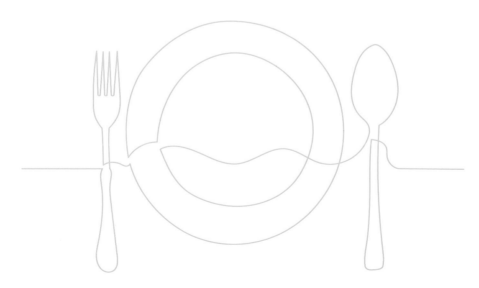

HOW TO USE THIS BOOK

Part 1, Transform Your Body, Mind, and Health, covers the basics of intermittent fasting, providing a comprehensive look at what intermittent fasting is and how it affects your body. You'll discover all the amazing physical and mental benefits of intermittent fasting. By the end of part 1, you'll be eager to get going.

Part 2, Get Started, sets you on your way, step by step, for successful intermittent fasts. The chapters in part 2 explain the best practices for each key stage of intermittent fasting: the fasting window, breaking the fast, and the eating window. You'll learn the best foods to eat (and the best ones to avoid), about supplements to support your progress, how to maximize your workout, and how to avoid the usual mistakes people make along the way. Each chapter includes a checklist to use to confirm you're on track with the essentials and a troubleshooting section to make sure you are fasting in a way that supports your body and lifestyle. Chapter 7 is your tool kit, including sample fasting schedules, to make your first step, or staying on the right path, even easier.

Part 3, Amplify Your Results, offers ways to kick your results into high gear by supercharging fat burning, crushing inflammation, and enhancing sleep. Because thyroid-related conditions and estrogen dominance are common challenges for many women, chapter 11 offers strategies for maintaining hormone balance as another means of optimizing the benefits of intermittent fasting.

Part 4, Make It a Lifestyle, shows you how to sustain intermittent fasting as a healthy living plan for the long term. You'll be able to maintain motivation through it all—hitting a plateau, mood swings, relapse—and bring your family along for the ride. If you take nothing else from this book, I want you to remember the message of chapter 14: Do what's best for you. This means listening to your body, honoring your goals, adapting as needed, and ignoring the haters. When you are fasting or practicing a healthy lifestyle, there will be people who say you're crazy, tell you that intermittent fasting is dangerous, and so on. Ignore them. This works. You know it (or will soon!) and the science backs up the results. For even more support and resources along the way, check out FastingIsEasy.com.

Ready to begin intermittent fasting and dramatically optimize your life?

Let's jump in.

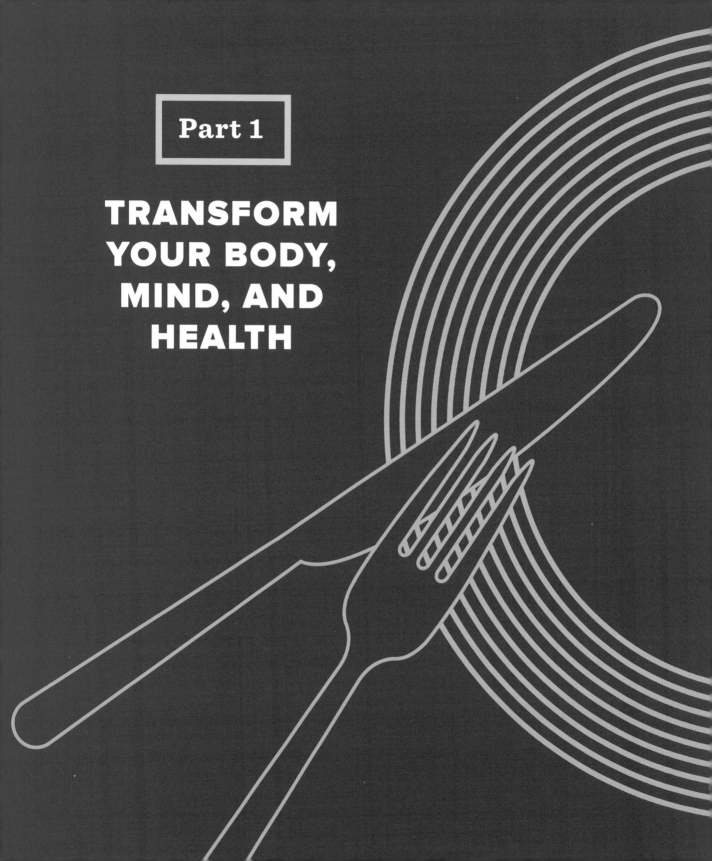

Part 1

TRANSFORM YOUR BODY, MIND, AND HEALTH

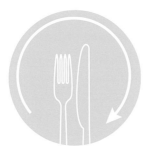

CHAPTER 1

What Is Intermittent Fasting?

Intermittent fasting is one of the most powerfully effective ways to get in shape and enhance your body, mind, and life. But, what exactly do I mean by *intermittent fasting*?

Simply, intermittent fasting is not eating for a set period of time, the fasting window, then consuming all of your daily calories during another set period of time, the eating window. For example, fasting (not eating) for sixteen hours of the day, then eating your daily meals during that remaining eight-hour window. It's about *when* you eat, not what you eat. Intermittent fasting meshes with any eating approach: keto, low-carb, paleo, vegan, vegetarian, whatever. In a nutshell: Intermittent fasting is a *meal-timing plan,* not a diet. That's basically it.

How can doing something so straightforward as not eating for a set period of time bring about an amazing array of benefits and transform your health? Fasting flips a metabolic switch that completely changes the way your body works. Flipping the switch alters the type of fuel the body uses—instead of running on glucose, the body starts running on fat—and sparks a host of physiological changes that go way beyond body composition to boost cellular rejuvenation, heart health, and brain function.[1] Fasting is not about restricting calories; it's about revealing a completely different side of our bodies, one we would never get to utilize unless we purposefully accessed it. Time to get excited about how your body works.

Intermittent fasting IS

✓ About flipping the metabolic switch to burn fat for fuel and optimizing the way your body works

✓ A meal-timing plan (*when* you eat)

✓ A set period of time per day when you do not eat followed by a finite period of time when you do eat

✓ Workable with any dietary eating style

Intermittent fasting IS NOT

✓ A diet (what you eat)

✓ Complicated (unless you want it to be!)

✓ Expensive

✓ Rigid or inflexible

YOUR BODY AND FOOD: WHAT HAPPENS WHEN YOU EAT

When you eat, your body goes into storage mode. Sure, some food we eat is converted into energy that's used right away, but most of us eat more than we need to, and what we don't need, we store.

Three macronutrients—carbohydrates, fat, and protein—are required in large amounts to provide the body with enough energy to function optimally. Each macronutrient has a unique part to play in the process.

→ **Carbohydrates:** Carbs are a quick and easily used energy source, which is why your body loves them. When you eat carbs, your body breaks them down immediately into a simple sugar called glucose, also often referred to as blood sugar. Glucose can be used instantly by all cells to power up, and any unused glucose is stored for later. There are two ways glucose is stored: First, it is stored as glycogen in the muscles and liver. Then, when the liver has reached its glycogen limit, excess glucose is packed away as fat in the liver and in adipose (fat) cells throughout the body. There is no limit to how much glucose can be reserved as fat.

→ **Fat:** The main fats in foods are triglycerides, made of three fatty acids and a backbone of glycerol. It takes a long time to break down and digest fats, which is why eating fat keeps us satisfied longer. These complex fat molecules provide the densest form of energy for your body, generating nine calories per fat gram compared to four calories in every carbohydrate or protein gram, but because the body prefers glucose, most fat isn't used right away for energy. Instead, excess fat is deposited in adipose cells.

→ **Protein:** Made of small units called amino acids, protein is critical for the growth and repair of virtually every cell and tissue in our bodies, from muscles and bones to skin and hair. Unlike carbs and fats, protein isn't a major go-to energy source, though under certain circumstances, it can be converted to glucose. The body can't store excess protein, so any extra protein eaten is converted to glucose and stored as glycogen or fat.

Eating

Storage Mode

High Insulin

**Glycogen and Fat Banked
for Later**

Insulin, made by the pancreas, is the hormone to watch when it comes to intermittent fasting. Its level in our bodies goes up when we eat, and a high insulin level keeps the body in fat-storage mode. Its level in our bodies goes down when we fast, and a low insulin level allows us to use stored body fat for fuel.

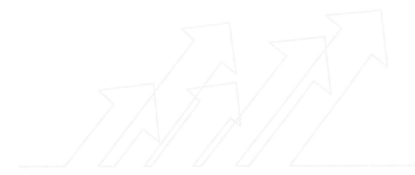

Ingesting any of these three macronutrients signals to your body that it's time to either use the food for energy immediately or, most likely, save it for later. One hormone is central to accomplishing both of these tasks: insulin.

Eating *any* type of food triggers an insulin response. This may surprise you: It's not just carbs that raise insulin levels. Protein and fat do, too. Although insulin is most well-known for shuttling glucose into cells for immediate use, it does the same for fat and amino acids.

But insulin isn't called an anabolic, or storage, hormone for nothing—any leftover carbs, fat, or glucose are stored as glycogen and fat by insulin. Insulin also keeps fat from being used as energy. Why start burning stored fat for fuel when food (more fuel) is coming in? High insulin levels promote fat storage and prevent fat burning.

When we eat and insulin levels remain high, we stay in fat-storage mode and don't tap into our energy reserves for fuel. The body runs on the incoming food (fuel) and packs away the leftovers—and unwanted pounds.

What if you could start using some of that fat for fuel instead? That's exactly what happens when we fast.

YOUR BODY AND FASTING: WHAT HAPPENS WHEN YOU FAST

When we are fasting, our bodies enter burning mode. Insulin levels go down, and so the body taps into glycogen, and then stored body fat, for fuel. When your body senses less energy coming in, it recognizes the need to flip the metabolic switch and start utilizing its stored fuel. That energy sensor is an enzyme called adenosine monophosphate-activated protein kinase (AMPK). When AMPK is triggered, it's like the low-fuel light going on in your car, telling you to get gas. That fuel light tells the brain that no food is coming in, so it's time to start burning stored energy.[2] When AMPK is activated, the move from fat-storage to fat-burning mode proceeds like this:

1. TAPPING INTO GLYCOGEN STORES. Once you stop eating and your body uses all the glucose in your bloodstream for fuel, insulin levels drop, and the body starts burning its fuel reserves. First up is glycogen, excess glucose stored in the liver.

2. BURNING FAT AND MAKING NEW GLUCOSE. With no new glucose coming in (because you aren't eating) and glycogen stores depleted, your body starts looking for other sources of energy. Triglycerides, the stored form of fat, are broken down into fatty acids that are released directly into the bloodstream. Just about every cell in the body can use fatty acids for fuel. Major exceptions to this rule are red blood cells and brain cells, which rely on glucose. To supply these cells and main-tain steady blood sugar levels—we still need stable blood sugar during a fast or we risk confusion, seizures, and death from hypoglycemia—the body starts manufacturing glucose from sources other than carbohydrates.

In a process called gluconeogenesis, glycerol from fat and amino acids from protein are turned into glucose in the liver.

(Wait. If amino acids from protein are being used to make glucose, does that mean you're losing muscle? Not so fast. A little later in this chapter, I'll cover how fasting does *not* cause muscle loss, and in chapter 2, I show how fasting helps build higher-quality muscle.)

When gluconeogenesis ramps up to produce glucose, the body also starts producing another energy source: ketones. When the liver breaks down fat, it uses the glycerol for gluconeogenesis and converts the remaining fatty acids to ketones, a very efficient fuel source that can power the brain.

3. RUNNING ON KETONES. Trying to run the body on glucose via gluconeogenesis is very costly. So, the body makes a shift, turning to ketones as the dominant energy source. Gluconeogenesis continues to happen—you still need glucose to survive—but ketones are now the body's primary fuel and are burned in a process called ketosis. Because making ketones relies on fatty acids, more ketone production means you're utilizing more fat for fuel. In this energy-burning phase, ketone production has nothing to do with being on a

No Food Coming In

Energy Sensor AMPK Triggered

Metabolic Master Switch Flipped

**Body Burns Stored Glycogen in
Liver and Body Fat for Fuel**

ketogenic diet and everything to do with your body switching to an alternative fuel source during a fast.

In addition to lowering insulin, fasting causes changes to several other hormones that also promote fat burning. These hormones are called counter-regulatory hormones because they run counter to insulin. When insulin levels go down, these hormone levels go up, and vice versa.

→ **High epinephrine (adrenaline) and nor-epinephrine (noradrenaline).** Fasting puts your body under a degree of stress, and that stress causes a big surge in the catecholamines epinephrine and norepinephrine.[3] These two hormones are the main drivers of fat burning and rev it up in a major way.

→ **High human growth hormone.** Secreted by the pituitary gland, human growth hormone preserves muscle, helps our bodies utilize fats better in an effort to save and spare our muscles, and prevents blood sugar levels from dropping too much by stimulating the liver to produce more glucose.[4]

→ **High cortisol.** This so-called "stress hor-mone" is not the enemy. It's a friend when you're in a fasted state. Here's what you need to know: Cortisol plays a dual role when it comes to fat. In the presence of food and insulin, cortisol promotes fat storage.[5] But, when we're fasting, it's a different ball game. Food is out of the equation and insulin is low. Now, spikes of cortisol free fat stores from the body to be burned for energy. Fasting leverages cortisol to your advantage. Keep in mind, cortisol levels naturally fluctuate, generally starting higher in the morning and falling throughout the day. Fasting doesn't chronically elevate our cortisol levels; rather, it makes the surges higher.[6]

When it comes to fasting, the sooner we tap into our energy reserves, the better. The goal of fasting, then, is to deplete glycogen stores and move into fat-burning mode as early in our fasting window as possible.

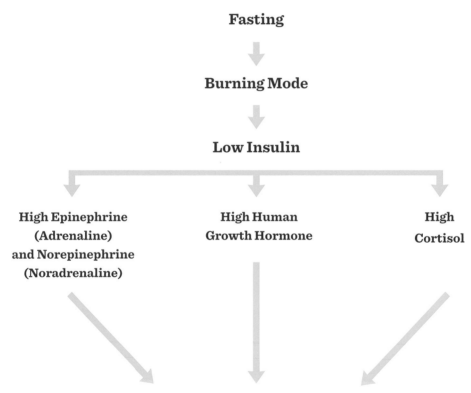

Fasting

↓

Burning Mode

↓

Low Insulin

High Epinephrine (Adrenaline) and Norepinephrine (Noradrenaline)

High Human Growth Hormone

High Cortisol

Glycogen and Fat Broken Down for Fuel

ANSWERS TO COMMON QUESTIONS ABOUT THE EFFECT OF FASTING ON THE BODY

There are a lot of myths and pieces of misinformation circulating about intermittent fasting. Let's clear the air on some of the most frequently asked questions.

Is intermittent fasting right for me?

I'm over age fifty.

You are not too old for intermittent fasting. Age alone (unless you are under 18, which means you should not fast until your body has fully developed) is not the determining factor as to how safe or effective intermittent fasting will be for you. Underlying medical conditions or medications may be an issue (see following entries), and it is a good idea to check with your health care provider before starting a fasting regimen. There are some steps you should take to make sure you are fasting in the healthiest and most effective way. Visit FastingIsEasy.com for more resources on how to fast safely over age fifty.

➜ **Ease into it.** Over age forty, we start to lose metabolic flexibility, the capacity to adapt easily to shifts in our diet. Similarly, your cells will take a little longer to get the hang of using stored energy substrates, such as fat.

➜ **Eat adequate protein.** As we age, we start to lose muscle mass naturally. To offset this loss, you need adequate protein on both fasting and nonfasting days. Aim for between two and three grams of protein per kilogram of body weight.

➜ **Support with supplements.** Supplements, such as vitamin D to further protect you from sarcopenia and age-related muscle loss, and coenzyme Q10 to support the ruthlessly efficient utilization of nutrients, will be an important part of your lifestyle.[7]

I have diabetes.

(If you have diabetes, or any type of condition, ask your doctor first before beginning.) In some, intermittent fasting has been shown to improve insulin sensitivity.[8] But, you will need to monitor your blood sugar and work closely with your health care provider to make sure your insulin and any other medications are properly tuned to ensure your blood sugar remains in a steady and proper range during your fasting and eating periods.

Fast with Caution If You . . .

✓ Have certain medical conditions (ask your doctor)

✓ Take medications

✓ Have a history of disordered eating

Avoid Intermittent Fasting If You Are . . .

✓ Under age 18

✓ Pregnant

✓ Breastfeeding

✓ Severely malnourished or underweight, with a body mass index (BMI) of less than 18.5

I have other medical conditions.

Speak to your health care provider before you begin fasting to make sure it is safe for you. Your health care provider's advice is especially important if you take medication, as some may be less effective or cause side effects if not taken with food.

I'm pregnant.

Fasting is not recommended during pregnancy. There isn't enough research on fasting's effect on pregnancy or the long-term effects that could appear later in the baby's life. Fasting may make it harder for you to get the proper nutrients you and your baby need and may alter your hormone levels in unpredictable ways. Why gamble?

I'm breastfeeding.

Fasting while breastfeeding is not recommended. If you're in any way nutrient deficient, your baby will be, too, and your milk supply may decrease. To avoid any risk of compromising your child's development, wait until your baby is weaned to start intermittent fasting.

I have a history of disordered eating.

Intermittent fasting should support a healthy lifestyle and quality of life. It is not a form of disordered eating, but if you find yourself so focused on fasting that your quality of life suffers or you develop a problematic relationship with food, such as severely restricting it, binge-eating, or guilt-driven purging, speak to a health care professional or counselor who can help you safely incorporate intermittent fasting into your lifestyle or find better ways to reach your health and wellness goals.

Will I lose muscle?

Fasting promotes muscle preservation and, if you do the right things after a fast, such as eat adequate protein and perform resistance training, can even help build higher-quality muscle. Although some protein is broken down during fasting, much of it is reallocated, not "lost." In one eight-week study, men ate and trained the same way, but one group fasted for sixteen hours per day whereas the other group did not. Both groups maintained all their muscle, but the fasting group lost significantly more fat.[9] Intermittent fasting does double duty, saving muscle *and* shedding body fat.

Your body has different needs while fasting. For example, it doesn't need amino acids and protein to build digestive enzymes during a fast. You're not eating, so why would you need digestive enzymes? Instead, those amino acids and protein can be reallocated where you do need them, such as supporting muscle preservation. So, it's all about reallocation.

We know this reallocation happens because autophagy, or the body's way of clearing out the old or damaged parts of cells and recycling them, increases.[10] Autophagy acts like Robin Hood, taking unnecessary or dysfunctional components from cells that are no longer needed, breaking them down, and supplying them to new areas of the body that could use a little extra support.

While autophagy works on reallocation, human growth hormone makes sure we're not breaking down protein and that the protein that is broken down gets used in the best possible way. *The Journal of Clinical Endocrinology & Metabolism* found that, even after a short fast, there was a five-fold increase in human growth hormone, and studies average a three- to five-fold increase.[11]

Researchers tested the protective power of all of this human growth hormone by giving somatostatin, which blocks growth hormone, to one set of study participants. Well, guess what happened when their protein levels were checked after a forty-hour fast? There was a 50 percent increase in the amount of protein excreted by the body in the participants whose growth hormone was inhibited compared to the control group. Meaning, when there was no growth hormone, protein wasn't being reallocated; it was being released en masse.[12] Elevated growth hormone levels during a fast help preserve muscle and lean body mass.

What this means is that you don't lose muscle while fasting. Any protein that's broken down from muscles is used elsewhere and, by clearing out and replacing the broken-down parts of your cells, you're setting the stage for better, stronger muscles.

Ketones produced when you're fasting also preserve muscle. In one study, researchers found that ketones reduced muscle breakdown by 18 to 41 percent.[13]

Will my metabolism slow down?

Fasting does not slow your metabolism, or basal metabolic rate (BMR), the amount of energy (calories) needed to perform basic bodily functions, such as breathing and circulation, at rest. Studies suggest fasting, instead, has a powerful effect on maintaining metabolism. One study found that twenty-four-hour alternate-day fasting (one day fasting, one day not fasting) for twenty-two days did not change the metabolic rate of participants, but they did lose weight.[14] I don't recommend this style of fasting long term, but these results highlight how fasting does not necessarily lead to a sluggish metabolism, and, in fact, research suggests it can cause the opposite, revving it up.[15] In one study, the metabolic rate increased on the first three days of a four-day fast.[16]

Your metabolism slows when the body tries to conserve energy. This often happens on calorie-restricting diets as the body responds to the scarcity of energy by lowering the rate at which it burns calories. During a fast, your body doesn't need to cut back on energy because it's able to tap into its fat stores and so has all the fuel it needs to keep everything humming. The rise in epinephrine and norepinephrine also stimulates your metabolism.[17]

Is intermittent fasting different for women?

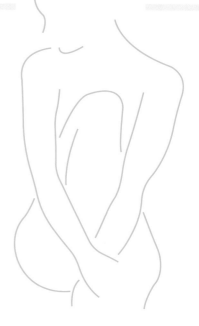

Fasting for women is not as different from fasting for men as you may think. The basics of how to fast and the benefits you will experience are essentially the same. That said, fasting puts stress on the body, and although stress isn't inherently bad and can lead to many positive outcomes, stress can also lead to negative hormonal changes, including to the reproductive hormones.

Much of the concern about women fasting relates to the hormone kisspeptin and its role in the menstrual cycle. Kisspeptin is very sensitive to fluctuations in insulin and other hunger-related hormones, in other words, fasting. The release of kisspeptin activates gonadotropin-releasing hormone, or GnRH, which, in turn, signals the pituitary gland to produce follicle-stimulating hormone (FSH) and luteinizing hormone (LH). FSH does exactly what it sounds like—stimulates the growth of follicles in the ovaries. LH tells the ovaries to release estrogen and progesterone and, during ovulation, an egg. Here's the issue: Some studies, such as one study done on fasting female rats (yes, rats, because of their similarity to humans anatomically, physiologically, and genetically), have found that kisspeptin and LH levels plummet.[18] Low levels of these hormones throw the body out of whack and could seriously compromise fertility. But the limited research is less than conclusive. Other studies done on women have shown little to no fluctuation in reproductive hormones.[19] What to make of this?

Listen to your body. Some women find they are more sensitive to the stress of fasting, especially in the week leading up to their period, when estrogen levels go down and increase their sensitivity to cortisol. If you find this is the case for you, scale back on your fasting schedule during that week. If you stop menstruating or feel like something is off in any way, stop fasting and contact your health care provider.

On the flip side, many women thrive with intermittent fasting, which should come as no surprise. The female body is designed to withstand longer periods of time without food as a way of protecting a potential fetus. It can weather the storm of a fast a bit better than the male body—and that can lead to some pretty awesome benefits.

On average, women have 6 to 11 percent more body fat than men,[20] and they have a higher percentage of fat than men of the same

WHAT IS INTERMITTENT FASTING?

Fasting Myth	Fasting Fact
✓ You'll lose muscle. ✓ Your metabolism will slow. ✓ Women shouldn't fast.	✓ You'll preserve muscle and be able to build higher-quality muscle. ✓ Your metabolism will not slow as your body has plenty of fuel from fat to supply all of its needs. Your metabolism is more likely to slow on a steady calorie-restricting diet. ✓ Women are uniquely designed to thrive with intermittent fasting.

weight, not only on their bodies but also within their muscles.[21] More fat is a benefit? Stay with me. Women are designed to use fat as a primary energy source and are better at utilizing it. In a fasted state, women kick-start the fat burning process sooner than men do. Plus, the epinephrine released during a fast is more potent in women, burning more fat than the same amount of epinephrine in men.[22] And during exercise, women use more fat for fuel while breaking down less protein.[23]

Although the essentials of intermittent fasting are the same for everyone, I recommend that women pay extra attention to their thyroid and estrogen because many women experience thyroid-related symptoms, such as hypothyroidism (underactive thyroid) often caused by autoimmune disease. To be clear, intermittent fasting has not been shown to harm the thyroid gland or significantly

change hormone thyroid levels, but because women are prone to thyroid-related issues, it makes sense to support the thyroid as much as you can.[24] I offer ways to do so throughout the book.

Estrogen dominance, a hormone imbalance in which levels of estrogen are high compared to progesterone, is also increasingly common among women of all ages, and I recommend ways to maintain a good balance in chapter 11. Estrogen affects much more than the menstrual cycle, including the brain, heart, and urinary tract, as well as bone, breast, and skin health. Keeping estrogen under control is critical for overall good health and to reap the maximum benefits from intermittent fasting.

HOW LONG TO FAST

There's no "perfect" fasting length, only the length that works for you, your body, your lifestyle, and your goals. Intermittent fasting is like the Swiss Army knife of wellness practices. You can use it in various ways to attain a range of results and goals. When deciding how long to fast, consider the following:

→ **Where you are on your intermittent fasting journey:** New to fasting? Start with a twelve-hour fast two or three times a week and increase the window up one hour each time, every week, until you hit a length that makes you feel good, energized, and upbeat. The idea is for intermittent fasting to become a lifestyle, which means making it sustainable. There's no point in jumping into a twenty-hour fast before you're ready and then feeling so cruddy you never want to fast again. Go at your own pace.

→ **Your goals:** Fat loss? Longevity? More energy and focus? Research tells us that certain fasting lengths support certain benefits, making it easy to tailor the length to best support your goal.

→ **Experimenting:** Don't hesitate to mix things up and evaluate how you feel after different fasting lengths, or even with different fasting lengths each week or month. I'm a big fan of cycling through different fasting times. Just remember the goal: to feel amazing, physically and mentally. Listen to your body. If you feel less than awesome, reduce the time and/ or frequency of your fast until you get to a good place.

→ **Individuality matters:** Your unique body, eating habits, and health history are significant factors that affect when you will experience certain benefits from fasting. The longer it takes to utilize your glucose and glycogen stores, the longer it takes to reach fat-burning mode. You may see benefits at sixteen hours that your best friend doesn't get until twenty hours. The following benchmarks are generalizations, meaning what happens in most cases. The recommendations in this book are geared toward getting you to the best possible results in the most efficient way.

Over time, frequent intermittent fasting results in less hunger. If you struggle with hunger as a major barrier to losing weight, you may find intermittent fasting helps you overcome that hurdle for good.[25]

Twelve-Hour Fasting Window/Twelve-Hour Eating Window

A twelve-hour fast is a good place to start if you're new to fasting or want to ease into it, testing the waters to see if it suits you. Benefits include:

→ **Gut microbiome reset.** An imbalanced and unhealthy gut microbiome overpopulated with "bad" bacteria is linked to digestive troubles, high blood sugar, and weight gain. A twelve-hour fast will help kill the bad bacteria and help rebalance your gut microbiome.[26]

→ **Food awareness.** There is a very powerful psychological effect that comes from a twelve-hour fast that should not be undervalued but is often overlooked: food awareness. So many of us don't eat with intention. We eat based on emotion, impulse, and stress. A twelve-hour fast gives you the opportunity to become more aware of when you eat and why you eat. Successfully doing a twelve-hour fast also gives you the confidence and discipline boost to take on longer fasts, when additional benefits kick in.

Sixteen-Hour Fasting Window/Eight-Hour Eating Window

This is one of the most common fasting schedules because it's where the magic really begins. After sixteen hours, AMPK has been activated and your body has likely switched from burning glucose and glycogen for fuel to burning fat.[27] You're continuing to starve the bad bacteria in your gut to reset your microbiome while also experiencing:

→ **Insulin vacation.** Once you approach the sixteen-hour fasting mark, you're giving your pancreas a break. Overproduction of insulin can lead to insulin resistance, which is when cells don't respond well to insulin and lose their ability to use glucose.

→ **Fat burning.** As insulin levels dive, gluconeogenesis ramps up to convert glycerol from fat into glucose. To feed that gluconeogenesis fire, you're burning more and more fat.

→ **Improved memory, focus, and brain function.** With the acceleration of gluconeogenesis comes increased ketone production and all its associated benefits.

→ **Longevity.** Autophagy, the body's recycling process, is clearing out the parts of cells that are weak and damaged, leaving you with stronger cells.

Eighteen- to Twenty-Hour Fasting Window/ Six- to Four-Hour Eating Window

Pushing a little past sixteen hours into the eighteen- to twenty-hour fasting window amplifies all the benefits of a sixteen-hour fast. The fat-burning fire that was lit at sixteen hours is still raging and blazing up even more of your fat stores. Ketone production increases and the difference can be substantial—in some studies, ketone levels doubled from fifteen to twenty hours.[28] Autophagy continues its cellular rejuvenation and anti-aging work.

Doing a twenty-hour fast brings more cellular rejuvenation and longevity benefits, especially by strengthening your cardiovascular system. Fasting for this length of time has been linked to an increase in vascular endothelial growth factor (VEGF), a signaling protein that promotes the growth of new blood vessels. Bonus: By increasing blood flow, VEGF also helps turn white adipose tissue, the fat you're probably most familiar with—typically in your hips, stomach, and thighs—and that stores extra energy, into the mitochondria-rich fat-burning brown adipose tissue. One more example of how fat burning is amplified.[29]

White Fat	Brown Fat
✓ Stores energy in large droplets throughout the body	✓ Stores energy in many smaller droplets, primarily around the neck, shoulders, and spinal cord
✓ Provides insulation	✓ Packed with mitochondria to burn fat and calories and generate heat
✓ Functions as an endocrine organ, releasing hormones responsible for regulating numerous functions throughout the body	✓ Linked to weight loss and improved blood sugar and insulin levels[30]
✓ Too much leads to obesity and a higher risk of developing certain chronic conditions	✓ Can be created from white fat in part by fasting for twenty hours

Find the Best Fasting Length for You

If You Want To . . .	Fasting Length
Begin a fasting regimen	12 hours
Increase your food awareness	12 hours
Reset and rebalance your gut	12+ hours
Boost brain function	16+ hours
Burn fat	16+ hours
Improve insulin sensitivity	16+ hours
Promote longevity	16+ hours
Optimize all the benefits of fasting	18 to 20 hours

HOW TO SCHEDULE YOUR FAST

Finding a fasting time frame that fits your lifestyle can be tricky. The good news is, there's a lot of flexibility here, and in the end, the choice is entirely yours. A few things to consider:

Your fasting window officially begins after the last bite of food enters your mouth.

Avoid eating after the sun goes down. This prescription means no late dinner before the start of your fast or breaking your fast at 10 p.m. Why? The body runs optimally when it's in sync with the circadian rhythm, the twenty-four-hour sleep-wake cycle regulated, in large part, by light and dark. Light triggers a hormonal cascade signaling the body to wake

up and be active, whereas darkness signals sleep and restorative mode. You might think that when you're asleep you're storing fat, but the opposite is true: You're more likely to burn fat at night because you're not consuming food. The body can't manufacture fat from thin air, after all. We need to give our body plenty of time in restorative mode, and that means when it's time to sleep, we should not be eating.

One recent study found that women who consumed their last meal between 7 p.m. and 7:30 p.m. lost almost 5 pounds (2.25 kg) more than those who consumed their last meal between 10:30 p.m. and 11 p.m., and they had lower fasting glucose levels, better triglyceride levels, and other key biomarker improvements.[31]

Living in sync with your circadian rhythm will have a positive effect on your metabolism and energy levels, helping you achieve better results all around. This schedule goes for fasting and nonfasting days.

Your preferred workout schedule.
To get the most benefit from fasting, you should work out toward the end of your fast.

Regarding fasting schedules, play around with timing. Don't be afraid to try a couple of schedules and mix them up throughout the week. It's good to keep your body guessing. Some fasting schedules to consider include:

→ **Beginning your fast after dinner, at 7 p.m.** Most people find that starting a fast after finishing dinner is a good way to go. This means eating your last meal of the day, fasting through the night while you sleep, and then breaking the fast in the afternoon or evening the following day, depending on how long your fasting window is. For example, a sixteen-hour fast with this schedule could mean beginning a fast at 7 p.m. and ending it at 11 a.m. the following day. This schedule basically has you skipping breakfast, which for a lot of people is pretty simple to do. Of course, extending your fast extends the fasting window into more of your day. Beginning a twenty-hour fast at 7 p.m. means breaking it at 3 p.m. You get the idea.

→ **Beginning your fast in the afternoon, at 4 p.m.** Skipping dinner can be more challenging for some, but this timing is a good way to stay in alignment with your circadian rhythm and fit in a workout in the morning. Starting the fast at 4 p.m. means you'd break a sixteen-hour fast at 8 a.m.

TOP TACTIC

Skip Dinner

Participants in one study who fasted for eighteen hours with a six-hour eating window from 8 a.m. to 2 p.m. showed lower levels of the "hunger hormone" ghrelin, decreased appetite and daily hunger swings, increased fat burning, and improved metabolic flexibility (the body's ability to switch between burning carbs and fats) compared to those who fasted for twelve hours with breakfast at 8 a.m. and dinner at 8 p.m.[32] Try eating earlier in the day and fasting in the afternoon and overnight.

HOW OFTEN TO FAST

I don't recommend fasting every day. It's called "intermittent" fasting because you are intended to fast at irregular intervals, not regularly, continuously, or steadily. The benefits of intermittent fasting come when it's done sporadically, shocking your body to make it better able to adapt to fat burning.

You may lose weight fasting every day simply because you're not taking in as many calories as you were before you started fasting but, eventually you'll hit a plateau. In a phenomenon known as adaptive thermogenesis, your body gets used to running on fewer calories and then lowers your metabolism, requiring you to either eat less and less to lose weight or exercise more and more for the same result.[33] Anyone who has ever tried to sustain weight loss by restricting calories knows all too well it's a dead end.

Calorie restriction is not the goal of intermittent fasting; flipping the body's metabolic switch, so the body becomes more efficient at burning glucose and fat for fuel, is. Rather than fast every day, fast smart and strategically to maintain its effectiveness and achieve the maximum benefit. Here's what I recommend:

Beginners: Fast two or three times per week.
Maximum: Fast three or four times per week.

That said, there is no hard and fast rule. Just as you'll experiment to find the fasting length that works best for you, try a variety of fasting schedules to find what best suits you. Monitor your results. Do you feel good? Are you seeing the results you want? Is your schedule sustainable? If you answered "no" to any of these questions, dial back your fasting schedule. Fasting too much will prevent you from reaping the maximum benefits.

LET'S BREAK IT DOWN

- Intermittent fasting is one of the most powerful ways to get in shape and enhance the heck out of your body, mind, and life.

- The basics are simple: Don't eat for a set period of time (the fasting window) and then consume all your daily calories during another set period of time (the eating window).

- When you eat, your body is in storage mode, banking excess macronutrients as glycogen and body fat.

- When you fast, your body is in burning mode, breaking down stored glycogen and body fat for fuel.

- Listen to your body and don't hesitate to try different fasting lengths and schedules until you find what works best for your lifestyle and that makes you feel physically and mentally energized.

- Keep the "intermittent" in "intermittent fasting"—don't fast every day.

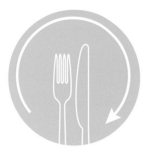

CHAPTER 2

Optimize Your Body

A lot of people associate intermittent fasting with changed body composition, and though those changes are significant, they are just the tip of the iceberg when it comes to the physical benefits of fasting. Not only can intermittent fasting burn fat and build muscle, but it may also slow aging, increase insulin sensitivity, reduce inflammation, improve heart health and vascular function, strengthen the immune system, support gut health, and boost energy. Fasting upgrades your body in powerful ways by changing how it functions at the cellular level, and there's a lot of exciting research to back up these claims.

A caveat: When you dig into the science of fasting, you notice something fairly quickly. Many studies are being done on animals—from flatworms to mice. Does that fact mean the findings are useless and misleading and should be discounted? No. Scientists wouldn't do these studies if they didn't believe the findings would be worthwhile, shedding light on how the human body works and how to apply the results to improve our health. Animals are biologically close to humans and mice, and humans share almost exactly the same set of genes, which means we have the same kinds of organs and similar circulatory, digestive, hormonal, nervous, and reproductive systems. So, although study findings on animals may not be one-for-one with humans, they can give a good indication of what could happen to the human body under similar conditions. Is it a guarantee? No.

So, why not just do these experiments on humans in the first place? Animals are much easier to control and monitor, ensuring that the experiments are handled exactly as intended and the findings are accurate. These animals also have shorter life spans, allowing scientists to measure the effects over the course of a life in a much shorter period of time than with humans. Say, 2 weeks rather than 100 years. The bottom line: We glean a lot from animal studies, but they have limitations we should recognize.

A wide range of research, on animals and humans, supports the many benefits of intermittent fasting. Don't take my word for it, though, or the words of all the scientists, either. Only you can decide if intermittent fasting is right for you and lives up to the promise of better health.

Top Body Benefits

Intermittent fasting can help upgrade your body by helping you:

✓ Lose weight

✓ Build muscle

✓ Gain longevity

✓ Increase insulin sensitivity

✓ Reduce inflammation

✓ Improve heart health and vascular function

✓ Strengthen your immune system

✓ Support gut health

✓ Boost your energy

WHAT THE SCIENCE SAYS

Intermittent fasting causes changes to your hormones, such as epinephrine and insulin, increases the efficiency of mitochondria, and changes the very nature of fat itself to maximize fat burning and utilization.

WHAT THIS MEANS FOR YOU

Intermittent fasting offers a proven weight-loss strategy that preserves muscle and does not slow your metabolism while also promoting significant fat loss.

Losing weight may be the primary reason you're interested in trying intermittent fasting, and if so, you're not alone. It helped me lose more than 100 pounds (45.3 kg), so I know it can help you look and feel your best. Weight loss is one of the most common reasons people try intermittent fasting because it is so effective at burning fat while preserving muscle—and that last part is important. You don't want to shed muscle; the more muscle you have, the more calories you can burn and the better able you'll be to sustain your weight loss by burning fat for fuel. Burning fat is what gives you the shift in body composition, and the changes to our cells' gene expression and hormones that occur due to fasting help us shed pounds while turning our bodies into efficient fat-burning machines that actually crave fat.

Fasting flips a metabolic switch in the body that initiates a cascade of hormone changes tied to the breakdown of body fat. Lower insulin levels allow fat burning. Spiking epinephrine activates hormone-sensitive lipase to start dumping massive amounts of stored fat into the bloodstream so we can utilize it.[1] Higher levels of human growth hormone inhibit the activity of lipoprotein lipase, the body's major fat-storing enzyme, reducing your body's ability to bank fat for later.

It's these hormonal changes—especially the effect fasting has on insulin—that distinguish intermittent fasting from other popular forms of weight loss, such as consistent calorie restriction. Studies comparing the two dietary approaches show both lead to weight loss, but fasting seems to reduce insulin to a greater extent.[2] If insulin levels remain high, the body never gets into fat-burning mode because high insulin equals fat storage.

But intermittent fasting doesn't just allow us to burn fat; it makes our bodies better at using fat for fuel. Fasting gives your cells a bigger net with which to catch fats circulating in the bloodstream and bring them into the cells for energy. That net is called CD36, a protein in the cell membrane that facilitates fatty acid uptake. Normally, you only have a little bit of CD36 expressed in the membrane, but AMPK activation signals a lot more to go to the membrane and start pulling fat into the cells[3]—and that fat is fast-tracked to the mitochondria. And, speaking of mitochondria, those energy powerhouses, fasting promotes mitochondrial biogenesis, the creation of new, upgraded, and more efficient mitochondria capable of burning more fat.[4]

Fasting even changes the way our fat operates. Exciting new studies are showing that during a fast, subcutaneous fat, the soft stuff you feel when you pinch the skin on your belly or thighs, turns into visceral fat. Wait: You may be wondering, isn't visceral fat, the fat stored deep within the abdomen surrounding vital organs, the "bad" fat, and all kinds of dangerous? Sure, we don't want too much visceral fat (or any fat), but we do want some to protect our organs and provide an immediate supply of energy. This transition from belly fat to visceral fat is a good thing because the body targets that visceral fat for burning *and* burns it six times faster than other types of fat.[5] You lose belly fat and visceral fat. Win-win.

You're also turning white fat, the kind with low blood flow that stores surplus energy and hormones, into brown fat—the kind of fat we want. Brown fat has much more blood flow and is packed with mitochondria to create energy and heat. How is this transformation possible? It comes down to an increase in vascular endothelial growth factor (VEGF) that triggers the growth of new blood cells in white fat.[6] Now, you have less white fat weighing you down and more brown fat filled with mitochondria using fat for fuel.

TOP TACTIC

Shrink Your Eating Window to Burn Fat

Simply by shrinking your eating window, you give the body a chance to use its stored fat for fuel. In one recent study, researchers compared two groups of men: one group on a daily sixteen-hour fasting window/eight-hour eating window and the other on a traditional twelve-hour eating pattern of three meals each day at 8:00 a.m., 1:00 p.m., and 8:00 p.m. Both groups ate the same number of calories and macronutrients and exercised in identical ways. The difference between these two groups came down to *when* they ate. After eight weeks, the intermittent fasting group had a 16 percent reduction in body fat versus a 2.8 percent reduction in body fat in the traditional-eating group with no change in muscle mass.[7] That's pretty amazing.

WHAT THE SCIENCE SAYS

Fasting increases human growth hormone and catecholamines, initiates autophagy, and improves insulin sensitivity to support higher-quality muscle building.

WHAT THIS MEANS FOR YOU

When it comes to building muscle, the food you eat to break your fast and the timing of your workout are even more important than the length of your fast.

In a fasted state, you have specific hormonal advantages, such as increased human growth hormone, to help preserve muscle, but does intermittent fasting promote muscle *building*? No, you won't magically gain muscle with fasting because growth hormone levels are elevated. Rather, fasting sets the stage for muscle building. Higher levels of human growth hormone play a part and so do raised catecholamines that increase blood flow to muscles. Cueing autophagy to break down weaker cell parts promotes muscle recovery and provides energy to the satellite cells that encourage the development of higher-quality muscle.[8] But, to gain muscle, you need to eat and work out appropriately to support its growth, and this is where insulin factors in.

When you're fasting and have gone a period of time without eating, your insulin levels lower and your body becomes more sensitive to insulin. So, when you do break your fast, your insulin levels spike in response. That's okay because there's nothing like a good, controlled insulin spike to help build muscle. A post-meal insulin rise activates the mechanistic target of rapamycin (mTOR), arguably the biggest driver of protein synthesis (the creation of muscle tissue from protein) and muscle growth.[9] Increasing insulin sensitivity by fasting flips mTOR into high gear. And, if you break your fast with a high-protein meal, your cells will have all the amino acids they need for muscle growth.

When you work out matters as much as how you break your fast. Exercise increases insulin sensitivity. By working out at the end of your fast, you take advantage of your already-improved insulin sensitivity and can further elevate protein synthesis when you break your fast post-workout.[10]

You'll find the precise steps and best practices for building muscle with intermittent fasting throughout this book.

PROMOTE LONGEVITY

WHAT THE SCIENCE SAYS

By activating the longevity gene FOXO3, PPAR-alpha, and autophagy, and enhancing telomerase activity, fasting helps support cell rejuvenation, regeneration, and overall health.

WHAT THIS MEANS FOR YOU

You have the potential to live longer and in better health.

Who doesn't want to look younger and be healthier while living longer? Fasting is a powerful rejuvenator from the inside out, improving your life span and your "health span," the amount of time you live in good health. You'll begin to see longevity-related benefits with sixteen-hour fasts, but the longer your fast, the greater the rewards.

The key to fasting and longevity? Using fat for fuel, and over time, becoming more efficient at processing fats. Utilizing fat for fuel affects your cells and genetic expression in several ways that may help you live longer.

Your FOXO3 gene is connected to life span and is commonly known as the "longevity gene." While you fast, the FOXO3 gene activity elevates dramatically to turn up cellular rejuvenation.[11]

If this gene were activated all the time, we'd probably live forever; it's that powerful. It's on when we're in a fasting state but turned off when we're in a fed state or storage mode.

Peroxisome proliferator-activated receptor alpha (PPAR-alpha) is a nuclear receptor, a class of proteins that turns genes on and off. It's activated when fatty acids are liberated from stored tissue and released into the bloodstream. Once mobilized, PPAR-alpha promotes the uptake and utilization of those fatty acids for fuel and the production of ketones, so we need it to get any of the benefits of a fast.[12] No wonder PPAR-alpha is referred to as "the key" to fasting. It may also be a key to slower aging. Research on animal models supports that PPAR-alpha signaling leads to better health and a longer life.[13] Studies on people suggest a direct correlation with increased life span. Individuals more than 100 years old—a good life span, I think we can agree—were found to have an upregulation of PPAR-alpha and clear signs of utilizing fats for fuel, such as high lipids in their blood.[14] All of this evidence suggests that when the body uses its own fat and PPAR-alpha is activated, there is a strong connection for improved overall longevity.

One reason cells are living longer and stronger is autophagy, the process that upcycles unwanted parts into energy or raw material for new growth. Think of autophagy as the survival of the fittest. Fasting creates a sort of scarcity effect within your body, which causes the body to double down and clear out what's not performing.[15] In this case, the malfunctioning parts of older, weaker cells are "eaten up" (*auto* means "self" and *phagy* means "eat," or "self-eating"), leaving you with only strong components and thriving, more efficient cells.[16]

When autophagy is on, mechanistic target of rapamycin (mTOR), the main driver of cell growth, is turned off, and when it comes to longevity, that's a good thing. Now, mTOR isn't "bad," we need cellular growth, and we don't want mTOR turned off all the time, but we also don't want mTOR activated all the time, either. A consistently high level of mTOR is associated with a shorter life span and even tumor growth. Periodic stretches where mTOR is turned off, and autophagy, essentially its opposite, is able to clean up like a janitorial crew, provide a balance beneficial to a longer life span.[17]

One type of cell that is more active and regenerative during fasting is stem cells, the body's raw material, capable of creating new, healthy cells to replace damaged ones. Fasting multiplies the stem cells that produce telomerase and enhances what's called telomerase activity. Telomeres are the protective structures at the end of chromosomes, the threadlike collection of your DNA. Each time a chromosome replicates, each time we activate our genes, the telomeres shorten. As those telomeres get shorter and shorter and shorter, we run the risk of a gene mutation that generates abnormal growth, dysfunctional cells, or short-lived cells. This is why short telomeres are linked to aging and the development of certain conditions. If we restore our telomere length, we could, essentially, live longer and remain healthier for an extended period of time.

Well, it just so happens that fasting activates telomerase, the enzyme that prevents telomeres from shrinking, and increases the number of stem cells able to produce telomerase.[18] More telomerase helps maintain the length of telomeres for longer periods and may even increase telomere length.[19] This extends life span and health span. Researchers studying young mice found that a calorie-restricted diet lowered the telomere shortening rate when compared to that of mice fed a normal diet, which led to a 20 percent increase in life span. Basically, their telomeres did not get shorter as fast as the other group did, and their life span was significantly longer.[20]

INCREASE INSULIN SENSITIVITY

WHAT THE SCIENCE SAYS

The prolonged periods of low insulin and fat burning associated with intermittent fasting improve insulin sensitivity and the efficient use of glucose.

WHAT THIS MEANS FOR YOU

A lower risk of insulin resistance and the serious health conditions associated with it, and a body that can process glucose more efficiently.

Insulin sensitivity refers to how responsive your cells are to insulin and, subsequently, how efficiently cells can absorb nutrients, such as glucose. If you're insulin sensitive, your cells readily absorb the sugar circulating in your bloodstream. The opposite of being insulin sensitive is being insulin resistant. In this case, cells can't hear insulin knocking on the door to usher glucose inside, resulting in elevated blood sugar, elevated insulin (the body keeps pumping out insulin, fruitlessly knocking even louder on the cell's door), and cells barking for energy but unable to access it. For example, people with type 2 diabetes are insulin resistant. Insulin resistance increases the risk for several serious health problems including heart attack, obesity, and stroke. It's estimated that one in three Americans is insulin resistant.[21]

We want to increase insulin sensitivity, so our cells become more receptive to glucose and other nutrients and use these nutrients more efficiently. With increased insulin sensitivity, your body can do a lot more with fewer carbohydrates, and fasting is one of the best ways to achieve this result.

Prolonged periods of low insulin levels improve sensitivity and, by now, you know insulin levels drop while fasting. Practicing intermittent fasting for twelve to sixteen hours resulted in a 25 percent decline, on average, of fasting insulin levels in one recent study.[22] This insulin level decline is the benefit of fasting versus regular calorie restriction. In one study comparing women who fasted two days each week versus those who reduced the number of calories consumed each day, both groups lost similar amounts of weight and fat, but the intermittent fasting group had tremendous improvements in their fasting glucose and insulin levels and insulin resistance.[23]

Reducing adipose tissue increases insulin sensitivity, and fasting has a significant capacity for fat burning and decreasing the amount of our body fat. When you fast for an extended period, accumulated fat deposits become the fuel that cells need to operate. As a result, the size of the excess fat droplets grows smaller over time. As the size of the lipid droplet in muscle and liver cells decreases, those cells become more responsive to insulin and the uptake of blood sugar and other nutrients, thereby increasing insulin sensitivity.

Fasting helps cells access glucose more easily and use it more effectively. When the body is in fat-burning mode, it casts a big net for energy. Just as it increases CD36 to catch fats, it hikes glucose transporter type 4 (GLUT4) to catch glucose from the bloodstream.[24] Remember, you need glucose; the body can't run on fats or ketones alone. In a fasted state, you become more efficient at using glucose as well as more insulin sensitive.

REDUCE INFLAMMATION

WHAT THE SCIENCE SAYS

By reducing body fat, improving gut function, initiating autophagy, reducing oxidative stress caused by free radicals, and stimulating the production of ketones, fasting is anti-inflammatory.

WHAT THIS MEANS FOR YOU

The benefits of overall reduced inflammation include a healthier immune system, increased energy, better muscle recovery and fat burning, and a lower risk of conditions associated with chronic inflammation.

Inflammation is essential for healing, but too much inflammation can be harmful. The redness and swelling that result after an injury help protect and heal, but when inflammation lingers and becomes chronic, the immune system gets overworked, trying to mend the area indefinitely, and white blood cells may even start attacking healthy tissue by mistake. Chronic inflammation is associated with a host of serious health conditions.[25]

Many of us have chronic low-grade inflammation caused by any number of reasons: environmental toxins, food sensitivities and allergies, poor sleep, stress, undiagnosed autoimmune conditions. Operating with chronic low-grade inflammation feels like you're running uphill all the time. You'll feel rundown and fatigued. Reduced inflammation is a major contributor to why many people feel more energized during a fast. Chronic inflammation puts your immune system on high alert 24/7 and that takes up a lot of energy, energy you may not even realize your body is using until you get it under control.

About 30 to 40 percent of American adults may have nonalcoholic fatty liver disease (NAFLD), a chronic condition in which excess fat is stored in the liver because the body is producing too much fat or isn't metabolizing it efficiently.[26] Researchers have found that when AMPK is activated, it may stop the storage of fat in the liver.[27] Another study showed that fasting changed the metabolism of fatty acids in the liver and improved glucose tolerance, the ability to process sugar.[28] In this way, intermittent fasting may help improve the functionality of your liver.

Reducing inflammation will also help you meet your fitness goals. Chronic inflammation steals energy that could be used for protein synthesis to build muscle, fat mobilization, and post-workout recovery. Every bit of muscle soreness is a result of inflammation, and if we prevent and reduce chronic inflammation levels, your body can use more energy to actually heal what needs to be healed.

Reducing inflammation often means dialing down an overactive immune system. This necessitates finding a delicate balance: We want to bring down inflammation just enough so we don't have chronic inflammation, but we don't want to bring it down too much, so we compromise our immune system by weakening it. Not fasting too long or too often, as well as breaking your fast in ways that support immune system recovery, are some ways I'll help you find that balance throughout this book.

Several benefits of fasting, such as reducing body fat and resetting the gut, are linked to reduced inflammation. By clearing out the damaged parts of cells, autophagy also reduces inflammation. Intermittent fasting enhances the body's ability to scavenge free radicals—unstable molecules that damage healthy cells and cause inflammation.[29]

In addition, ketones are anti-inflammatory. When you're fasting and gluconeogenesis has been initiated, you are producing ketone bodies. These ketone bodies suppress inflammation. A study from Yale School of Medicine found that exposing human immune cells to the ketone beta-hydroxybutyrate (BHB) following two days of fasting resulted in a significantly reduced inflammatory response.[30] The ketones worked by countering a set of proteins (called the NLRP3 inflammasome) that triggers inflammation: no more rogue proteins triggering inflammation, taking energy from building muscle or burning fat.

We know the effect fasting has on inflammation because we can track several testable markers. Monocytes, a type of white blood cell, are largely associated with chronic inflammation. A nineteen-hour fast reduced the circulating levels of monocytes and, therefore, resulted in less inflammation.[31] That's really great news—but it gets better. Not only are fewer monocytes being pulled from the bone marrow and released into the bloodstream, but the ones that are being recruited release fewer inflammatory cytokines. Fewer circulating monocytes potentially means you have less ability to fight infection during your fasting period, but it's definitely a good thing to fight chronic inflammation. It's all about finding the right balance and not crushing your immune system too much or when you are especially vulnerable.

Remember that study (see page 39) that found shrinking the eating window to eight hours resulted in a significant reduction in fat compared to a traditional eating style? It also showed a significant reduction of inflammation levels.[32] The fasting group had a massive reduction in tumor necrosis factor-alpha (TNF-α) and interleukin 1 (IL-1), two cytokines or cellular messengers that drive inflammation. Fasting changed body composition and it stimulated a healthy recovery.

IMPROVE HEART HEALTH AND VASCULAR FUNCTION

WHAT THE SCIENCE SAYS

The body's switch to burning fat for fuel stops the creation of new triglycerides and LDL cholesterol, while elevating vascular-supporting ketones and improving heart rate variability (HRV).

WHAT THIS MEANS FOR YOU

A happier, healthier heart.

We know lifestyle matters when it comes to improving heart health. Fasting has been demonstrated to improve several factors involved in heart health, including blood pressure, triglyceride and LDL cholesterol, and resilience to stress.[33]

Lower levels of triglycerides and LDL, low-density lipoprotein, or "bad" cholesterol, makes sense because triglyceride levels affect those of LDL. Here's how: When the liver's glycogen stores are full, excess glucose is converted into triglycerides and released as very low–density lipoprotein (VLDL). VLDL is transformed into LDL. Well, once you stop eating, glucose is no longer coming in, the metabolic switch is flipped, and the liver stops making new triglycerides.[34] Triglyceride levels decrease because you're not forming new ones. In one study, triglyceride levels dropped by 32 percent after eight weeks of alternate-day fasting.[35] No new triglycerides means no VLDL being released and no new LDL, lowering those levels, too.[36] The same study noted a drop in LDL of 25 percent.[37]

Heart rate variability (HRV) is a way to measure resilience and parasympathetic tone, or how well your body is able to switch between the sympathetic (fight-or-flight) and parasympathetic (rest-and-digest) nervous systems. HRV measures the variation in time between heartbeats. If you're stressed, the variation between heartbeats is low. If you're more relaxed, the variation is high. A low HRV is associated with an increased risk of heart conditions.[38] Intermittent fasting has been shown to increase your HRV by putting your parasympathetic nervous system in control.[39]

In addition, beta-hydroxybutyrate, the main ketone body, improves the integrity of vascular cell walls, the inner lining of arteries, capillaries, and veins. Safeguarding these walls is essential for a healthy cardiovascular system.[40]

WHAT THE SCIENCE SAYS

Fasting restocks white blood cells and revamps memory T cells to remodel the immune system.

WHAT THIS MEANS FOR YOU

Amplified ability to prevent and fight illness over the long term.

Fasting helps your body fight invaders, but it's not a one-time, quick immune stimulator. It's not a good idea to fast when you're worried about getting sick because, during the fast, especially longer fasts, your immune system is somewhat suppressed. Key circulating immune system cells that fight bacteria, viruses, and other invaders, such as monocytes and T cells, decrease.[41] These decreased levels can compromise the body's ability to fight acute infection. However, over the long haul, fasting gives your immune system a solid benefit, essentially remodeling it into a more powerful one.

It's about finding balance: on the one hand, timing your fasts properly and not fasting so often or so long that you crush your immune system too much, and on the other, fasting enough so that you can enjoy the immune-boosting benefits.

The reduction of inflammation and microbiome and gut support that occur with fasting promote a stronger immune system. A huge portion of your immune system is located in your gut—around 70 percent.[42] Giving your gut a chance to heal is one of the most meaningful ways to improve immunity.

But, fasting can actually remodel your immune system. When you fast for a few days, your white blood cell count goes down—one study found that a three-day fast resulted in a 28 percent decrease. Those white blood cell count levels were restored when the fast ended. Why? Fasting kick-starts stem cells into regeneration mode, increasing the production of white blood cells to replenish the immune system.[43] A refreshed and renewed pool of white blood cells essentially refreshes and renews the entire system.

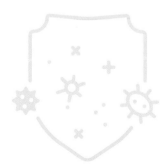

Memory T cells "remember" pathogens, making it easier for them to target and neutralize those pathogens if they appear in the body again. While you are fasting, memory T cells decline, which at first sounds bad, but stay with me. Researchers found that memory T cells rehome in the bone marrow where they get stronger and their "memory" improves.[44] These "Immune System Special Forces" troops return to base recharged, so when the fast ends, they come back fiercer and better able to fight invaders.

WHAT THE SCIENCE SAYS

Fasting promotes the die off of "bad" bacteria in the gut microbiome, and the ketones produced during ketogenesis in a fasting state improve our gut stem cells' ability to regenerate.[45]

WHAT THIS MEANS FOR YOU

A total gut reset leading to better digestion and nutrient absorption, plus the increased ability to fight infection and other invaders due to a stronger immune system. Your gut lining has a chance to heal, preventing toxins from entering your bloodstream and your immune system from having to ramp up and fight those nasties all the time.

Researchers have been paying increasing attention to the gut, and for good reason. A healthy gut goes way beyond good digestive health, though let's not underestimate less bloating, constipation, diarrhea, gas, and other common forms of gut distress. About 70 percent of the immune system is located in the gut. By restoring gut health, the immune system improves, too.

The gut has millions of neurons, more than are located in the human spine. Those neurons are known as the "second brain," or enteric nervous system. The gut and brain are in constant communication via the vagus nerve—the gut-brain axis—which explains why your stomach hurts when you're worried. In addition to running the digestion show, this second brain influences your mood. About 90 percent of the body's serotonin, the "happy hormone" that reduces anxiety and tension and stimulates feelings of well-being and happiness, is produced in the gut.

The gut also has a pretty big effect on your ability to burn fat. Researchers have found that the changes to the gut microbiome caused by fasting promote converting white fat into brown fat, a transformation that increases the number of mitochondria in the tissue and ramps up fat and calorie burning.[46]

There are two main ways gut health becomes compromised: gut dysbiosis, an unbalanced gut microbiome lacking diversity, and leaky gut, when the lining of the intestine becomes "leaky," allowing partially digested food, bacteria, and toxins to seep into the bloodstream.

Fasting resets the gut microbiome, the trillions of bacteria and other microbes that live in the intestines, by promoting the growth of good bacteria while flushing out and killing bad ones. This happens in a few ways. Raising immunoglobulin A (IgA) heightens our immune system's response and promotes the colonization of good bacteria, a protective mechanism when the body is stressed.[47] IgA also heightens the immune response of the gut mucosal lining, strengthening the buffer that keeps unhealthy bacteria from getting into the intestines. Mice on an alternate-day fasting schedule were able to clear salmonella bacteria out of their system more than twice as fast as the nonfasting infected mice.[48] The bacteria just moved right through their system without being absorbed. Finally, fasting starves bad bacteria, most of which have a high rate of doubling, and so are ravenously hungry all the time. Without enough food, the bad bacteria die, clearing the way for good bacteria to multiply.

The gut mucosal layer acts as a barrier, keeping partially digested food and bacteria inside the intestines and pathogens out. If the tight junctions maintaining the integrity of the mucosal layer weaken, harmful substances leak into the bloodstream and stimulate an immune system response. This increase in gut permeability, or "leaky gut," leads to chronic inflammation. In a vicious cycle, leaky gut is often caused by chronic inflammation. Fasting improves the stability and structure of the gut mucosal lining by dramatically improving intestinal stem cells' ability to regenerate. Intestinal stem cells are responsible for maintaining the integrity of the gut lining and repairing any damage. Researchers found that stem cells from fasting mice doubled their regenerative capacity.[49]

Taking a break from digestion gives your gut a chance to heal and clean house. The housekeeping crew within your gut can't do its job until food is out of the system. Better to clean an office after all the employees have left, right? Same with your gut.

BOOST ENERGY

WHAT THE SCIENCE SAYS

Fasting improves the efficiency of mitochondria, the cell's energy powerhouse, requiring less fuel to generate more energy.[50]

WHAT THIS MEANS FOR YOU

No mid-morning slumps or late-day sleepiness; enough get-up-and-go to do everything on your to-do list and then some.

The busy lives we lead can sap our energy, leaving us exhausted and unmotivated. Fasting offers a natural, long-term energy lift.

Reduced inflammation is one reason for the energy increase, but fasting increases the density and efficiency of the mitochondria, the energy powerhouses inside our cells, upping the amount of energy each can hold. Your body improves at building a better factory to house energy.[51] That fact alone will boost energy, but fasting also improves the efficiency of the mitochondria, increasing how much energy we can produce with less fuel. One landmark study on rats found that their heart increased energy output by 24 percent, with significantly less oxygen coming in, when they were in a fasting state and had ketones in their body.[52] Remember, your body starts making ketones when you've run through your glycogen stores and you're making glucose through the process of gluconeogenesis. Ketones burn cleaner than glucose, so as a result, you generate more energy with less fuel. Your body is like a car running on significantly less gas, but still able to generate more horsepower and torque.

When you feel drained, a lack of good sleep is often the culprit. While fasting, you should wake up feeling perfectly recharged because the quality of your sleep is improving. Participants in a study of healthy, non-obese volunteers were found to wake up less frequently and have less leg movement during sleep when they were in a fasted state, resulting in better concentration and emotional balance during the day.[53] Upgraded sleep while fasting is likely due to how quickly your body shuts down when your head hits the pillow. When you're awake while fasting, your sympathetic nervous system, the part that activates the fight-or-flight response, is turned on because fasting is a type of stress. Your blood pressure and heart rate are up. Your body is on alert. But the moment you lay your head on the pillow, your body shuts down hard to conserve precious resources. Your parasympathetic nervous system slows everything, ushering in rest, relaxation, and restorative sleep.

You know, now, that fasting improves gut health, but you may not realize just how much that digestive relief will increase your energy. Whenever we eat, we have anywhere from a 25 percent to 200 percent increase in blood flow to our guts.[54] Think about that. That's a lot of energy! When we take a break from eating and digestion, we can use all that energy elsewhere. Plus, by healing our guts so our immune systems don't have to fight toxins leaking into our bloodstreams continuously, we increase our vitality.

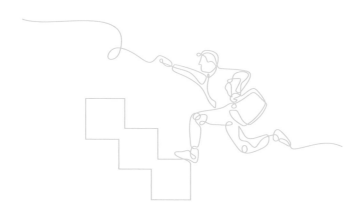

LET'S BREAK IT DOWN

- The potential physical benefits of intermittent fasting go far beyond the most frequently talked-about body composition improvements, such as fat loss.

- Intermittent fasting is linked to increased insulin sensitivity and lower inflammation.

- Being in a fasted state powers up the body's utilization of fat for fuel and autophagy, a process that upcycles unwanted cell parts, both associated with longer life spans.

- Immediately following a fast, your gut mucosal layer is a little weaker, but your microbiome is shifting and improving, and, over time, the stability and structure of the gut lining improves as intestinal stem cells increase their capacity to regenerate.

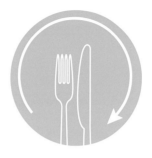

CHAPTER 3

Optimize Your Mind

Fasting is a powerful way to support your brain. It sparks the recycling of old cells, the protection of existing ones, and the growth of entirely new ones. That's right. By not eating for a period of time, you provide your brain with the fertilizer it needs to upgrade, so you can stay sharp now and as the years progress.

While you're fasting, your body goes into survival mode, and that's a *good* thing for your brain. A lot of energy gets diverted to the brain so it can be hyperfocused on the task at hand. From an evolutionary standpoint, this allocation of energy makes perfect sense. Our brain is our best, strongest tool when it comes to survival—it gives us an edge.

We need brains, not our brawn, so our bodies reallocate resources to keep the brain running optimally. The result? The brain boosts its abilities during a fast. Brain fog clears and mental clarity, focus, and productivity soar. But the benefits to the brain extend beyond the fast itself. Fasting may protect against cognitive decline.

IMPROVE COGNITIVE FUNCTION

WHAT THE SCIENCE SAYS

Fasting increases brain-derived neurotrophic factor (BDNF), improving brain neuroplasticity, so our brain uses energy better, increasing GLUT3 to fuel more shuttle buses of energy reaching the brain and increasing the number of mitochondria in the brain and its capacity to produce energy.

WHAT THIS MEANS FOR YOU

A big brain benefit. Not only is your brain using fuel more efficiently, but it's also getting more fuel, boosting your brainpower, and sharpening your concentration, thinking, and problem-solving skills.

An abundance of research supports the variety of ways fasting is good for your brain. In one study, fasting aging male rats showed improvement in cognition, learning, memory, and motor coordination as well as increased brain activity and growth.[1] In another study, mice on an extended alternate-day fasting schedule improved their ability to acquire and integrate new information.[2] Human studies tell a similar story, countering the notion that going without food leads to compromised thinking, recall, and reasoning. After a twenty-four-hour fast, women showed no impairments when it came to sustained attention, attentional focus, simple reaction time, and immediate memory.[3] And even after two days of fasting in a double-blind, placebo-controlled crossover study, participants exhibited no negative effects when it came to cognitive performance and activity, not to mention sleep and mood.[4]

If you've ever done a bout of intermittent fasting, you know how crystal clear your brain feels and how "in the zone" you can be when you need to be (and if you haven't yet tried intermittent fasting, get ready!). That increased focus happens because fasting boosts brain-derived neurotrophic factor (BDNF), a protein that supports the growth of neurons, the nerve cells in the brain that transmit information through electrical and chemical signals. A study published in the *Journal of Neurochemistry* found that stints of intermittent fasting for just a few weeks could improve BDNF levels anywhere from 50 percent all the way to 400 percent.[5] That's pretty incredible, especially when you consider how powerful BDNF is. We used to think that once you lost brain cells, you lost them for good, but now we know that's not true. BDNF enables our brains to produce new brain cells, and even preserves existing cells. BDNF keeps our brain cells from dying while also supporting new growth in the hippocampus, cortex, and basal forebrain, the parts of the brain that regulate memory, learning, and higher cognitive

TOP BRAIN BENEFITS

Intermittent fasting can facilitate a brain
upgrade by helping you:

✓ Improve cognitive function

✓ Elevate mood

✓ Encourage self-knowledge and self-mastery

function. And, this benefit goes even further by promoting synaptic plasticity, the ability of synapses to strengthen or weaken over time.

Synapses are the gaps between neurons that allow them to talk to each other via chemical or electrical signals and send messages throughout the body. How effectively neurons communicate with each other is controlled by the strength or weakness of these connections. Don't think of strong as good and weak as bad, though. Think of the way neurons speak to each other as a dialogue, and sometimes the neurons need to shout to be heard (a strong connection) whereas other times, a whisper (a weak connection) will suffice. Synaptic plasticity is the ability to adjust as needed. Without this adaptability, neurons can't transmit information well and messages get garbled, dropped, or lost. This prevents critical neurotransmitters, such as dopamine, norepinephrine, and serotonin, from doing their jobs and compromises learning and memory. BDNF makes the conversations between neurons rise and fall smoothly.

All of this new growth, the creation of new neurons, and the new neural connections that go along with them, plus the promotion of synaptic plasticity, contribute to neuroplasticity, the brain's ability to change and adapt—essentially to shape-shift. Neuroplasticity is linked to strengthening overall brain fitness, enhanced cognitive function, and better memory.

BDNF also helps the brain use energy better by upregulating GLUT3, so you get more shuttle buses delivering glucose to the brain.[6] Pumping up the energy even further, BDNF

TOP TACTIC

FAST FOR PEAK BRAIN PERFORMANCE

You get a big cognitive boost while fasting, so if you know you need to be at your best for a long day of meetings or an important presentation, plan to fast. The last thing you want is to be fatigued and foggy when the stakes are high!

swells the number of mitochondria within the brain. More of these energy powerhouses means the ability to produce more energy, specifically in the brain, to support focus and learning.

BDNF does a tremendous job helping your brain operate at its absolute cognitive best while you're fasting, but fasting's effect carries long afterward, too. Fasting protects brain cells from injury and prevents degeneration. Overall, low levels of BDNF are linked to cognitive impairment and memory loss, so the hike we get in BDNF from fasting shouldn't be minimized.[8]

Ketones, the substances produced when your body switches from burning glucose to burning fat for energy, may be at the root of elevated BDNF as they act directly on nerve cells to upregulate BDNF.[9] But, ketones are high-octane brain fuel in their own right. Beta-hydroxybutyrate (BHB), the main ketone body, is able to cross the protective blood-brain barrier and provide the brain with the most efficient source of energy possible—BHB releases 27 percent more Gibbs free energy, the amount of energy available for work, compared to glucose—an energy source your brain doesn't usually have access to.[10] This increased access to energy for the brain means improved focus and concentration, sharper thinking and mental acuity, and better memory. But ketones have also been found to increase the number of mitochondria, or "energy factories," in the brain cells of the hippocampus, a part of the brain important for learning and memory.[11] As powerful anti-oxidants, ketones offer long-term benefits by removing free radicals, a major source of stress on brain cells that are capable of wrecking their structure. High levels of free radicals are linked to aging and neurodegeneration.[12]

The more we can support brain health, the better off we'll be. At a time when dementia is a global epidemic and almost 5.5 million Americans have Alzheimer's disease—one new case is diagnosed every four seconds—and nearly one million are living with Parkinson's disease, protecting our brains against degeneration should be a priority for everyone.[13]

The upregulation of autophagy strengthens and protects cells throughout your body by upcycling old and dysfunctional parts, but in the brain, autophagy has been shown to defend against the buildup of amyloid plaques thought to destroy synaptic connections in areas of the brain connected to memory and cognitive function.[14]

By reducing inflammation, fasting also lowers the risk of neurodegenerative decline/damage. Chronic neuroinflammation is associated with many chronic conditions, resulting from the decay and death of neurons. A 2015 study on rats looking at neurodegenerative damage linked to inflammation found that intermittent fasting reduced the risk of damage to brain function.[15]

When we think of improving insulin sensitivity, we often think of decreasing our likelihood of becoming insulin resistant and developing an inability to lose weight, but what if it also played a part in reducing the risk of neurodegenerative damage? Insulin resistance happens all over your body, including your brain, and research suggests that brain insulin resistance contributes to the atrophy and demise of nerve cells.[16]

INTERMITTENT FASTING MADE EASY

ELEVATE MOOD

WHAT THE SCIENCE SAYS

Elevated BDNF has an antidepressive effect on the body and supports neuroplasticity for better, more stable moods while raising serotonin, the happy chemical.

WHAT THIS MEANS FOR YOU

A brighter, more stable mood and improved overall emotional well-being with fewer symptoms of anxiety and depression.

Fasting elevates your mood and makes modulating your moods easier. Fasting is also linked to fewer signs of depression, and because it has a positive impact on serotonin levels, you should feel calmer, emotionally stable, happier, and more focused.

Mood problems have been associated with low BDNF and synaptic plasticity. The elevated levels of BDNF that occur while one is fasting have a powerful antidepressive effect within the body. Significant decreases in anger, confusion, tension, and total mood disturbance and improvements in vigor were found in a study of aging men on an intermittent fasting regimen for three months.[17]

Remember, synapses allow neurotransmitters to do their thing. When we have synaptic plasticity, we can modulate our moods more easily. For example, we're able to strengthen or weaken a synapse whenever possible, like turning up or lowering the volume on the conversation between neurons. Now, you might be wondering, "Why would I want to weaken a synapse?" Well, you don't want a constant surge of serotonin, right? When you're scared or frightened, you wouldn't want the feel-good chemical pumping. You want to be frightened, because that feeling allows you to do what you need to do to get out of harm's way.

Or you don't want that synaptic volume turned way up for dopamine when you're touching a hot stove. Dopamine is your reward system, so why would you want to signal to your brain that it feels good to touch a hot stove?

Sometimes, we want a weak synapse and sometimes we want a strong synapse, and by fasting and raising BDNF, we're able to promote that modulation better. That's exactly why this ability is called synaptic plasticity. We have now made our synapses more flexible, allowing us to be more flexible in our moods. We're better able to control how we feel and adapt much better to stress. While you fast, you may notice you have the ability to turn your brain on and off really fast. Higher BDNF and synaptic plasticity is one reason for this ability.

Additionally, there's a pretty cool reciprocal arrangement between BDNF and serotonin, the feel-good neurotransmitter with an outsize role in regulating mood and your overall sense of well-being. Fasting increases BDNF, and BDNF increases serotonin, and serotonin signaling within the body increases BDNF expression.

One study tracking BDNF and serotonin levels in individuals fasting from sunrise to sunset during the month of Ramadan found significant increases in both.[18] After fourteen days of intermittent fasting, BDNF levels increased by 25 percent, and at the end of the study, after twenty-nine days, it had increased 47 percent. When it came to serotonin, the results were even better. After just fourteen days of fasting, there was a 33 percent increase in serotonin levels, and after twenty-nine days, researchers found a 43 percent increase. More serotonin helps you feel happier and calmer during your fast, and by elevating both of these chemicals, our overall levels of BDNF skyrocket over time and crystallize these positive mood-supporting brain changes.

Anxiety and depression have also been linked to inflammation. By decreasing body fat, improving gut function, initiating autophagy, reducing oxidative stress caused by free radicals, and stimulating the production of ketones, fasting reduces inflammation to prevent or ease these conditions. One study took a deep dive into the connection between fasting and anxiety and found that, after a twenty-four-hour fast, mice had a 40 percent reduction in anxiety-like behaviors and a 31 percent increase in their object location memory, their ability to find an object.[19] Fasting prompted an improvement in anxiety

symptoms *and* memory. Anecdotally, that rings true as, I don't know about you, but if I'm anxious or suffering from anxiety, my memory goes out the window.

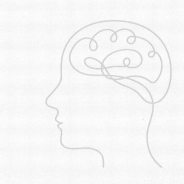

Ketones have been shown to lower stress and anxiety levels by helping facilitate the conversion of glutamate, an excitatory neurotransmitter that fires neurons into action, to GABA, an inhibitory neurotransmitter that produces a calming effect by blocking certain signals. A study published in the journal *Trends in Neurosciences* showed that ketones directly inhibited the ability of neurons in the hippocampus section of the brain to "load up" on glutamate while increasing the amount of GABA.[20]

TRUE OR FALSE?
BEING HAPPY AND FEELING GOOD
HELPS YOU BURN FAT

True!

Serotonin is far more than a one-trick pony making you feel upbeat and relaxed. It also helps liberate fat from storage and releases it into the bloodstream to be used as fuel.[21] So, not only does serotonin help us burn fat, but it also drives up the amount of fuel we have available to burn.

ENCOURAGE SELF-KNOWLEDGE AND SELF-MASTERY

Two elements essential to becoming the best version of yourself are self-knowledge and self-mastery, and these are two of my favorite benefits of fasting.

You will learn a lot about yourself and your body while fasting. It's a great way to become more aware of why you eat and when you eat. Boredom? Habit? Impulse? Routine? Or, to achieve nutrition and health goals? Taking a pause from eating and digesting gives you the chance to use that energy elsewhere and reconnect with your goals and motivation for achieving them. You'll also be more in tune with what your body is telling you—before, during, and after a fast. The goal of fasting is to feel your absolute best, physically and mentally. Holding firm to this goal offers an opportunity to give focused attention to what we're really feeling and give our body more of what it needs to feel great and make adjustments along the way—to fasting length, timing, the means of breaking a fast, or whether we fast at all—to achieve our goals.

This leads me to self-mastery, also known as self-discipline or self-control. We live in a world of instant gratification—if we want something, we can have it delivered practically the same day. If we want to feel good about ourselves, we're just an Instagram post away from a bunch of likes that will validate us. Rewards come at warp speed and they're killing our self-discipline, that perseverance, that grit, to achieve success that requires long-term commitment. Health and fitness goals require a long view. One workout isn't going to give you abs of steel any more than eating a handful of blueberries will eliminate your chronic inflammation or one sixteen-hour fast will zap your middle-aged middle. When we focus on short-term rewards, we weaken our capacity to achieve those rewards that require persistence. Intermittent fasting challenges our ability to delay gratification and bolsters our self-mastery, so we can actually attain the health and fitness we want. It reminds us that we are in control of how we reach our goals. In a world where you can't control a lot of what's coming at you, it's nice to know you can control what you put into your mouth and when. Delaying gratification until your eating window opens provides a sense of satisfaction that comes from taking another successful step on your health journey. That good feeling is magnified a thousandfold when you, ultimately, reach your destination. Trust me.

Knowing I'm capable of remaining focused on the task at hand and saying "no" to distractions has helped in many ways. That said, self-mastery can be taken too far. If you find that intermittent fasting triggers increased rigidity and obsession, bingeing behaviors, or disordered eating in any way, seek professional help.

LET'S BREAK IT DOWN

- Fasting is very, very good for your brain, providing immediate benefits, such as renewed mental clarity, focus, and productivity during a fast, and long-term benefits, including protection against cognitive decline.

- An increase in brain-derived neurotrophic factor (BDNF) is just one reason intermittent fasting provides such a brain boost. More ketones, less inflammation, the upregulation of autophagy, and better insulin resistance improve brain function and protect the brain against degeneration.

- Fasting elevates your mood and makes modulating your moods easier. Fasting is also linked to fewer signs of depression, and because it has a positive impact on serotonin levels, you should feel calmer, more focused and emotionally stable, and happier.

- Intermittent fasting reconnects you with your body and your health and wellness goals, fostering self-knowledge and self-mastery.

Part 2

GET STARTED

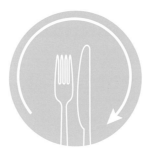

CHAPTER 4

Your Fasting Window

The benefits of fasting only come when you're in a fasted state, and although fasting is pretty simple—don't eat—there are nuances to it that frequently trip people up and ruin their progress. In this chapter, you'll find out how to get into a fasted state as quickly as possible, stay in it for the length of your fast, and avoid the most common mistakes that will unwittingly mess you up.

DECIDED ON THE LENGTH OF YOUR FAST?

SELECTED WHEN YOU'LL BEGIN YOUR FASTING WINDOW?

Good. (If not, return to pages 28–34 in chapter 1 for help determining the best fasting length and schedule for you.) Now, let's jump into everything you should and shouldn't do to get the maximum benefit from your fast.

During your fasting window, you want to avoid doing anything that will spike your insulin levels (remember, high amounts of insulin cause your body to store fat, not burn it) or trigger a metabolic response in your body. Most foods and drinks with a caloric value and/or an ingredient that raises insulin will kick you out of a fasted state. This means as close to zero calories as possible coming in. I grant amnesty to some things with a few calories because they won't have a significant effect on your fast and many have attributes that can actually help it. These exceptions include herbal tea and dried spices, especially turmeric and ginger. On the flip side, I recommend avoiding certain foods that have zero calories (looking at you, artificial sweeteners) because of their overall negative effect, especially on the gut. It's not about living according to a textbook; it's about living in a way that will get us to our desired outcome.

You have to ask: What is your end goal? Is it to obey the fasting police and feel good because you followed the perfect protocol, or is it to get results? I'm for results.

If You're Looking for Rigid, Look Elsewhere

I'm not a dietician or doctor, and I don't pretend to be. When I recommend foods to eat, I'm not rigid when it comes to the specific amounts or portion sizes. I may suggest "a little" of this or a "moderate" amount of that—even if I do provide a specific measurement, don't consider it gospel. This is going to frustrate some people who like exactitude, but I want you to be empowered to find your own way, using my suggestions as guidelines. There's no one-size-fits-all here, and that's a good thing. Should you feel overstuffed going into a fast (or ever, really)? No. Lean on my advice, use your best judgment, and embrace the experiment.

And, when it comes to supplements, follow the Recommended Dietary Allowance (RDA), or work with your health care provider to identify the proper type and dosage for you.

BEFORE YOUR FASTING WINDOW
WHAT TO EAT AND DRINK

What you eat leading into a fast makes a big difference in results. We want to move the body into a fasting state as quickly as possible so you experience the most benefit from the fast. That means your pre-fast meal should be modest in size (no giant meals before a fast), easy to digest, and able to send the proper signals to put you in fasting mode most quickly. The best way to do this is to keep the foods high in fat and as low in carbs as possible.

→ **High fat.** Most foods contain a mixture of different fats but are often higher in one kind of fat than others.

Saturated fats, generally solid at room temperature and often sourced from animals, such as butter and red meat but also found in coconut oil, are slower to digest.

Unsaturated fats move through the digestive system fairly quickly. Both monounsaturated and polyunsaturated fats are usually liquid at room temperature and are found in avocados, fish, olive oil, and walnuts.

I recommend choosing a high-quality fatty fish before a fast. Think: anchovies, mackerel, sardines, and sockeye salmon. These foods are easy to digest and rich in omega-3 fats, a polyunsaturated fatty acid and potent activator of PPAR-alpha, the "key" to fasting that gives our genes the go-ahead to start using fat for fuel.[1]

Vegans and vegetarians can get their fats by adding a little avocado oil (or a slice of avo),

coconut oil, MCT oil, or olive oil to tempeh, or coconut oil or MCT oil to a hemp or pea protein shake.

→ **Low carb.** Carbohydrates spike insulin, and high insulin prevents fat burning. But we also know now that carbs elevate the hormone leptin.[2] Leptin is good because it stimulates metabolism, but it has to be present in low levels for fat burning to occur.[3] By keeping carbs low, we tap into the body's fat-burning potential earlier in the fast.

→ **Modest amount of fiber-rich veggies.** A ton of veggies is going to slow your digestion, but a small amount that is high in fiber, such as ½ to ¾ cup (weight varies) of dark leafy greens (28 g to 41 g) or broccoli (36 g to 53 g), will break down into short chain fatty acids. These chemicals signal the brain to utilize fats better, and one short chain fatty acid, butyrate, can actually spur the production of ketones![4]

→ **Season with Mediterranean herbs.** When combined with foods containing high amounts of omega-3 fatty acids, oregano, rosemary, sage, and thyme all switch on PPAR-alpha.[5] Use fresh or dried herbs or an extract. If you prefer to lean into one herb, go with rosemary, as it activates PPAR-alpha via two different mechanisms.

→ **Apple cider vinegar.** To kick-start digestion, drink a little bit of apple cider vinegar. I like to make mine a "lemonade" by mixing it with some water, a squirt of fresh lemon juice, and a dash of cayenne pepper. Add a bit of stevia or monk fruit for sweetness.

Once the last bit of food from your pre-fast meal passes your lips, your fasting window begins.

What does my "perfect" pre-fast meal look like?

✓ Sockeye salmon seasoned with oregano, rosemary, sage, and thyme and cooked in (or drizzled with) extra-virgin olive oil or avocado oil

✓ Dark leafy greens

✓ Apple cider lemonade

WHILE FASTING: WHAT TO EAT AND AVOID

Let's get rid of the guesswork and start seeing results.

What to Eat and Drink

→ **Water.** Staying hydrated is of key importance while fasting. Drink plenty of plain sparkling (club soda or seltzer) or still tap or mineral water. Flavoring the water with a lemon or lime slice (or squirt of fresh juice), a piece of raw ginger, or the dried spices listed in this section is fine. Lemon and lime juice will help clear your digestive system and expedite the fast and gut healing.[6]

→ **Coffee without creamer, artificial or sugar alcohol sweeteners, or fats added, or flavored coffee (hazelnut, caramel).** Black coffee with nothing added to it is okay to have. I think coffee is one of the best things to consume while you fast. Yes, it has a few calories, but the net effect on your fast is positive, and that's what we want.

Caffeine triggers the body to burn more fat by stopping the inactivation of cyclic adenosine monophosphate (cAMP).[7] If cAMP is blocked, the body can't tap into stored energy. Caffeine makes sure cAMP is open for business, giving your body access to those fat reserves. Both caffeinated and decaf coffee are rich in polyphenols, compounds that act as antioxidants, reduce inflammation, and drive autophagy.[8]

So, don't be afraid of black coffee, but don't go overboard with four, five, or more cups, or have a cup too close to the end of your fast. Caffeine raises cortisol, and we don't want a pulse of cortisol right before we break our fast and pulse our insulin. Remember, cortisol is not inherently bad; it stimulates fat loss. But, elevated cortisol in the presence of high insulin can result in fat storage.

If your coffee is bitter without anything added, you need better coffee. It's worth the investment. Or try cold brew. I don't really like the taste of coffee, but I can drink cold brew without any problem. The "natural flavors" in most flavored coffees could be pretty much anything, so play it safe and avoid them.

→ **Tea without creamer or artificial or sugar alcohol sweeteners.** Black, green (including matcha), herbal, oolong, pu'er, and white teas flavored with lemon, lime, or dried spices (if desired) are okay.

Green tea is my favorite beverage during a fast. I usually sip on it throughout the fasting window. The caffeine is a fat mobilizer, and green tea helps activate AMPK, the fuel sensor that tells the brain to start burning stored fuel for energy.[9] Green tea also contains the phytonutrient EGCG, which can help inhibit the breakdown of your body's natural fat-burning catecholamines, epinephrine and norepinephrine, so they last longer.[10] Plus, green tea is great for the gut. And, although we know that fasting ultimately restores and strengthens the gut, some gut breakdown occurs during the actual fast. Drinking green tea before your fast will give your gut extra support. Recent research on mice suggests the villi, the finger-like projections that stick out from the small intestine and absorb nutrients, atrophy during a fast, but drinking green tea before and during fasting prevents this breakdown. Additional research shows that green tea also wards off the breakdown of the gut mucosal layer.[11]

One more reason I am such a fan of green tea: It promotes calm, relaxation, clear thinking, and long-lasting energy without the jitters.

I've also started sipping on lemon verbena tea throughout my fast, as it activates PPAR-alpha and helps drive me deeper into a fast.[12]

→ **Natural sweeteners, such as stevia (pure or liquid) and monk fruit.** If you must use a sweetener, these are your best options, though I advise you to go easy—or skip them altogether. Powdered stevia contains maltodextrin, a filler that will cause an insulin spike, so opt for pure stevia or the liquid version instead.

→ **Electrolytes.** These minerals conduct electricity when dissolved in water and are essential for many processes throughout the body, including maintaining proper nerve and muscle function, internal pH levels, and hydration. Electrolytes can become significantly depleted during a fast because, when we

produce less insulin, our kidneys release more sodium, potassium, and magnesium.

Sodium. We can lose anywhere from 23 to 345 mg of sodium per day of fasting.[13] Sprinkle high-quality salt, such as pink Himalayan salt or Celtic sea salt, into your water or other beverage to increase sodium levels. Sodium is important for maintaining adequate blood volume so we have enough blood to deliver waste to the liver, where it's processed and excreted during our fast. Salt also helps us retain precious water, fight fatigue, and feel satiated. We crave sweets when we're deficient in salt. Start with ¼ teaspoon of salt per half gallon (2 L) of liquid and see how you feel. You should feel a little energized. If you feel sluggish, then you don't need the additional salt and should stop supplementing with it.

If you're over age forty, you may need more sodium, up to 1 teaspoon per half gallon (2 L) of liquid.

Potassium. Early in a fasting state, we can lose 500 to 600 mg of potassium.[14] Low potassium leads to poor nerve signaling, which makes you feel tired and as though your muscles just aren't working right. Adequate potassium allows you to contract your muscles more and, potentially, burn more fat.

Magnesium. Magnesium is involved in more than 350 different enzymatic processes in the body, and most of us are deficient in this mineral. Even though we don't lose as much magnesium as sodium and potassium (studies suggest a rough average of 80 to 200 mg per day), I think we have the highest risk of depletion because we're starting in need.[15] During a fast, magnesium keeps electrolyte levels stable and produces energy. And magnesium provides the best of both worlds—relaxing the muscles and mind without lessening the effect of epinephrine when it comes to heart rate and lipid utilization.[16]

→ **Water-soluble vitamins and supplements.** Most vitamins and supplements are designed to make things easier on our bodies, but that's not what we're going for during a fast. We want to make things a little difficult so our bodies adapt and come back stronger. For example, vitamin C has been shown to "protect" the body during a fast, which negates the benefits (the stress of fasting helps your body become stronger, and the antioxidant effect of vitamin C shields the body from experiencing the stress).[17] That said, water-soluble vitamins, such as vitamin C and B-complex vitamins, won't break a fast, but some cause nausea when taken on an empty stomach. I recommend saving your supplements for your eating window and focusing, instead, on replenishing electrolytes during your fast.

→ **Apple cider vinegar.** Drinking apple cider vinegar during your fast will help kick you into a fasted state a little more quickly by triggering AMPK, the energy sensor that tells the body to start using stored energy.[18] It enhances fat loss by upregulating PPAR-alpha and initiating the gene expression we need for fatty acid oxidation.[19] The acetic acid in apple cider vinegar supports the microbiome, among its other digestive benefits.[20] I like to drink it

TOP TACTIC

DRINK THIS TO GET YOU OVER THE MID-FAST HUMP

Combine, to taste:

- ✓ Apple cider vinegar
- ✓ Cream of tartar (1 teaspoon = 495 mg potassium)
- ✓ Fresh lime juice
- ✓ Monk fruit (optional)
- ✓ Salt

before I go to bed or first thing in the morning. Sometimes I'll drink it straight, and other times I'll make a lemonade with a dash of cayenne pepper, ginger, or turmeric.

→ **Dried spices and herbs.** Add these flavor enhancers in powdered form to beverages for added flavor and to put you deeper into your fast. Yes, they contain a couple of calories, but the benefits far outweigh them.

Ginger. Ginger increases the effectiveness of a fast in several awesome ways. It triggers fat to leave cells and enter the bloodstream, signaling PPAR-alpha to turn on our fat-burning genes.[21] Ginger also spikes epinephrine, allowing you to oxidize and use fat for fuel.[22]

So, here we have ginger mobilizing fat and activating the genes and process, which allows us to burn fat. It gets even better. The two main compounds in ginger, gingerols and shogaols, allow your body to accumulate cAMP, a signaling molecule inside cells that increases the potential to burn fat.[23] Ginger's effectiveness increases when paired with caffeine, so ginger plus coffee or tea can be extremely powerful. I mix dried ginger into my green tea and water throughout my fast.

Cayenne pepper. I'm a big fan of starting my day with a bit of cayenne because the capsaicin it contains raises epinephrine and kick-starts the metabolic processes we need to get into a fasted state.[24] I sprinkle it in apple cider vinegar.

Turmeric. By elevating cAMP, the curcumin in turmeric flips on the AMPK energy sensor to initiate the metabolic change to fasting mode and gets autophagy going.[25] It also cues autophagy through an entirely different pathway, by activating transcription factor EB (TFEB), giving you two powerful ways to reset your body.[26] Combining curcumin with exercise increases mitochondrial biogenesis, the creation of new and improved mitochondria capable of burning more fat.[27] Spice up a beverage with a little bit of turmeric, about ½ teaspoon in water or other approved-for-fasting beverage.

Cinnamon. Cinnamon mimics insulin within the body and can help lower blood sugar, getting you into a fasted state more quickly.[28] Cinnamon is especially beneficial toward the end of your fast, when we want to control insulin before eating.

→ **Adaptogens.** Herbs or medicinal mushroom extracts, adaptogens help us manage stress better by promoting balance. I find the enhanced mental benefits of adding ashwagandha, Lion's mane, maca, reishi, or rhodiola rosea to my coffee outweigh the few calories added. You can also drink them brewed as a tea.

What to Avoid

→ **Food.** Seems obvious, but no food. Don't assume beverages, because they are liquid, aren't food. They may contain carbs, fillers, preservatives, protein, and so on that can break your fast or lessen its effectiveness.

→ **Coconut water.** Although it is hydrating, coconut water contains a fair bit of sugar, about 1 to 1.5 grams of sugar per ounce (30 ml), and that will definitely spike your insulin.

→ **Fats,** such as butter, coconut oil, essential oils (peppermint, lemon), ghee, and MCT oil. Fats are fuel, and by fasting, we're trying to use our stored fats. Consuming fats, even just adding them to beverages, will break your fast and put a buffer in front of the stored fuel you're trying to use up.

MCT oil. Medium chain triglyceride (MCT) oil is touted for its many benefits—and rightly so. It has thermogenic properties that help you burn more fat and can be converted to ketones for a high-voltage source of energy.

But it is fuel, and it will break your fast. Consume it—and coconut oil, a natural source of MCT—during your eating window only.

Bulletproof coffee. Bulletproof coffee, made with high-quality fats such as MCT oil and ghee, is phenomenal if you're on a keto diet. But it does not lend itself to fasting. Do you know how many calories are in one cup? We're talking 300, sometimes 400, calories. That's a lot of calories and is not, in any way, fasting safe. Drink bulletproof coffee *after* your fast.

→ **Protein powder.** This food item will definitely break a fast.

→ **Sweeteners, artificial and sugar alcohols.** *Artificial sweeteners, such as aspartame (Equal), saccharin, and sucralose.* Though these sweeteners may not cause a significant insulin spike or, technically, break a fast, I don't think they're worth the risk because of the negative effect they may have on your gut microbiome. More research is needed, given the conflicting findings, but I suggest avoiding these products.[29] Keep in mind, the commercial version of sucralose, Splenda, is cut with dextrose and/or maltodextrin, bulking agents that are, essentially, glucose, which will clearly break a fast.

Sugar alcohols, such as xylitol and sorbitol. Most sugar alcohols stimulate a digestive system response because about 50 percent of the amount consumed is absorbed by the small intestine.[30] Erythritol is the exception, not seeming to affect serum levels of glucose or insulin or negatively impact gut bacteria.[31]

Sugar Alcohols: Beware the Bloat

When ingested, sugar alcohols are incompletely absorbed, sending some to the bloodstream, while the rest passes through the small intestine and into the large intestine, or colon. The undigested amounts sit in the colon, ferment, and can cause bloating, gas, and even diarrhea. This doesn't happen to everyone; some people are more sensitive than others.

→ **Products that contain artificial and/or sugar alcohol sweeteners.**
Flavored water, diet sodas, energy drinks, and other beverages. Be wary of flavored and diet beverages as they often contain sweeteners plus lots of other ingredients, fillers, preservatives, and additives that won't do your fast any favors. Keep it simple and stick with plain water, coffee, or tea flavored with a little lemon or dried spices.

Gum. I'm okay with the few calories from gum if it doesn't contain artificial sweeteners or sugar alcohols, but that can be a challenge to find. Chewing gum may also make you hungry, exactly what you don't want. Best to avoid it altogether.

Mints. Even if you can find a breath mint with natural sweeteners, mints have more body, calories, and volume than gum. Say no to mints.

Toothpaste. Most toothpastes contain sweeteners, such as sodium saccharin, sorbitol, and xylitol. Also, watch out for fluoride as it can spike insulin.[32] Best to avoid these or make a concerted effort to rinse and spit thoroughly after brushing to avoid swallowing any toothpaste.

Mouthwash. It is often sweetened with saccharin.

→ **Cream, creamers, milk, milk substitutes.** All of these dairy and dairylike items have significant calories. Just stay away from them during your fasting window.

→ **Bone broth.** Containing calories, collagen, and protein, bone broth (and broth in general) is a food with a metabolic effect on the body. It has a place after your fast but not during it.

→ **Fat-soluble and soft-gel vitamins/supplements.** Avoid all supplements in this capsule form—a thin gelatin shell filled with liquid. These capsules contain fat and oil, both of which will break a fast. Common supplements in this form are fish oil and vitamins A, D, E, and K.

→ **Antioxidants.** Antioxidants are a big no-no during your fast because they hamper the metabolic and immune boosting effects of the fast. Adding antioxidants, such as vitamins C and E, blunts your body's ability to develop its own antioxidants.[33] Let the fast strengthen your immune system, and skip the antioxidants.

TOP TACTIC

MAKE YOUR OWN PRE-WORKOUT SUPPLEMENT

Make a fasting-safe pre-workout supplement by combining beta-alanine and citrulline malate. Beta-alanine buffers the burning feeling you experience while working out, allowing you to push it more. Studies have shown that the time to exhaustion can improve by ten to thirteen times.[34] Citrulline malate increases blood flow and fat mobilization to help your workout overall.

Start with 200 to 300 mg of each and work your way up to 1,000 mg of each. Beta-alanine can make you feel tingly, which is totally normal; just don't overdo it. I like to mix 1,000 mg of beta-alanine and 5,000 mg of citrulline malate with coffee for an energy boost and to make my workout seem easier. Researchers have found that, on average, coffee reduces the rating of perceived exertion by 5.6 percent.[35] I'll take that!

Most multivitamins contain antioxidants, so avoid those while fasting.

→ **Probiotics.** Let your gut rest naturally during a fast and save the probiotics for your eating window.

→ **Pre-workout supplements.** Most pre-workout supplements contain fillers, flavors, and other ingredients, such as maltodextrin, which will trigger an insulin spike or otherwise compromise the fast.

→ **BCAAs** (branched-chain amino acids). These contain leucine, an amino acid that triggers beta cells within the pancreas to secrete insulin and activates mTOR, the main driver of cell growth.[36] This is exactly what we don't want to happen during a fast. At their very core, BCAAs are the opposite of fasting.

→ **Alcohol.** Alcohol contains seven calories per gram, which means there is a strong metabolic response within the body to process alcohol. It will break a fast.

→ **Tobacco.** Smoking won't break a fast, but you know it's bad for your body any time, right? Chewing tobacco will definitely break a fast because of the amount you ingest.

→ **Vaping.** The nicotine ingested while vaping won't break a fast, but the sugars and additives in the flavorings might.

TOP TACTIC

FOR WOMEN AND PEOPLE OVER FORTY: CONTROL YOUR CAFFEINE

Women: Caffeine boosts autophagy and cell rejuvenation, which are good things, but women are more sensitive to caffeine, and too much will stress your body to the point where your hormonal cycles could be thrown off. Limit caffeine and choose lower or no-caffeine coffee and tea options, such as oolong or ginseng tea.

People over forty: Drink caffeinated beverages in the morning, a few hours after waking, then wean yourself off them over the course of the day. As we age, we're more susceptible to catecholamines, which are already surging in higher spikes during a fast, and consistently elevating them with caffeine will leave you exhausted.

Should I Have This During My Fast?

Yes	No
✓ Adaptogens	✗ Alcohol
✓ Apple cider vinegar	✗ Antioxidants
✓ Cayenne pepper, ground	✗ Artificial sweeteners
✓ Cinnamon, ground	✗ BCAAs
✓ Coffee, plain	✗ Bone broth
✓ Electrolytes	✗ Bulletproof coffee
✓ Ginger, raw, sliced (for flavoring) or ground	✗ Coconut water
✓ Lemon, slice or squirt of fresh juice	✗ Cream and creamers
✓ Lime, slice or squirt of fresh juice	✗ Fats
✓ Natural sweeteners	✗ Fat-soluble and soft-gel supplements
✓ Tea, plain	✗ Food
✓ Turmeric, ground	✗ Milk and milk substitutes
✓ Water, plain still or sparkling	✗ Multivitamins
✓ Water-soluble vitamins*	✗ Pre-workout supplements
	✗ Probiotics
	✗ Protein powder
	✗ Sugar alcohols
	✗ Tobacco
	✗ Vapes

*Remember, antioxidants are in the "no" column, and that means no vitamin C.

HOW TO WORK OUT

You should absolutely work out in a fasted state. If I hadn't trained while fasting, I don't think I would have been able to lose 100 pounds (45.3 kg) as quickly as I did. Why?

→ **More fat loss.** When you work out in a fasted state, you recruit intramyocellular lipids, droplets of fat stored in your muscle cells, and burn them two to three times faster, sometimes even more, than in a nonfasted state. You mobilize and use more fatty acids for fuel, and, over time, your body becomes more efficient at using them.[37]

→ **Increased insulin sensitivity.** Training in a fasted state turns up the dial on the energy sensor AMPK by 25 percent to improve insulin sensitivity.[38] Even when you're not fasting, your body is better able to use carbs and doesn't need as much glucose to get the job done. So, by training while fasted, you become efficiently dual-fueled, like a hybrid car, giving you an advantage over nonfasting trained individuals.[39]

→ **Improved muscle recovery.** After a workout, glycogen uptake in the muscles increases, giving you more energy for your next workout.[40]

→ **Better muscle building.** Increased insulin sensitivity and protein synthesis help you build muscle post-workout.

→ **More autophagy.** Exercise, especially cardio, amplifies autophagy.[41]

And the list goes on. Working out during your fasting window has so many advantages, it's really a no brainer to do so. If you want results, work out on an empty stomach. You don't necessarily need to change your workout routine; just remember this: Always exercise during your fasting window.

Don't baby your workout because you're fasting, but don't feel you have to push it during a fast, either. Keep it light, or at the intensity level from which your body can recover easily. You're getting more out of your workout just being in a fasted state.

Strength Training

Don't skimp on strength training—you'll use lots of fat and maintain your muscle mass while doing it. One study found that weight training during caloric restriction ended up accounting for a 93 percent preservation of lean muscle mass.[42] Basically, simply by touching a weight when you're fasting, you're going to preserve almost all of your muscle. *Everyone* should aim to preserve muscle. If building muscle is your endgame, pairing fasted strength training with proper protein intake post-fast is a great way to go.

Strength training during a fast activates localized mTOR, the primary driver of protein synthesis and muscle building. When mTOR is on, you're building muscle; when mTOR is off, you're not. Fasting turns off mTOR. During a fast, the body isn't in building mode; it's in recycling mode driven by autophagy. But it turns out that just the mere act of making your muscles work against a weight or force—doing some curls or squat thrusts—activates mTOR at the muscular level.[43] Protein synthesis turns on in the muscle while it's off everywhere else. That helps preserve muscle while still giving you all of the cell upcycling of autophagy. It's amazing. Even more amazing is that mTOR remains elevated at that muscular level for twenty-four hours.[44] *Twenty-four hours.*

That ongoing protein synthesis means you don't need to eat immediately after your workout to get the muscle-building benefits. You don't need to replenish your protein right away. So, don't break your fast early because you think you need to eat immediately after your workout. Get your workout in and carry on with the rest of your fast.

If you're looking to build muscle, you'll have a better result working out toward the end of your fast. You can capitalize on the insulin sensitivity from the fast itself and the increase in sensitivity from your workout. This way, you'll have a bigger insulin spike when you do break your fast. Higher levels of insulin equal higher levels of muscle building.

Cardio

If your focus is losing weight, cardio is an excellent way to torch fat. Train early in your fast, or in the morning when you have a little bit more in your tank, and benefit from all the fat burning that will continue after your workout and throughout the rest of your day and the fast.

High-Intensity Interval Training

A combination of strength training and cardio, high-intensity interval training (HIIT) is a good way to burn fat and preserve muscle. You do need some calories after a HIIT session, so I recommend training toward the end of a fast so you can break the fast soon afterward. For example, if I plan to break my fast at noon, I'd start my HIIT workout at 11 a.m.

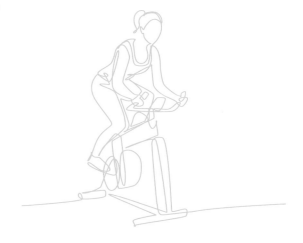

Plan a yoga session during your fast; it's great for fat loss and mood. In one study, women who took thirty yoga classes over twelve weeks saw a significant reduction in waist circumference and decreases in BMI, total weight, and body fat percentage.[45] In contrast, self-esteem went up! Larger studies have shown similar results. So, get on your mat!

There's no better way to become discouraged about intermittent fasting than thinking you're doing everything right, only to have one or two little things throw a wrench in your efforts. To get the most benefit from fasting, or to stay in a fasted state, avoid these mistakes.

→ **Eating something that compromises the fast's effectiveness.** This is hands down the most common mistake beginners make. The biggest culprits are:

- ✓ BCCAs
- ✓ Creamers, milk, and dairy substitutes
- ✓ Supplements, such as fish oil and vitamin C
- ✓ Sweeteners

→ **Not hydrating enough.** Hydrate, hydrate, hydrate. Your body needs adequate water to run. Period. And, during a fast, it's even more important to support your body with adequate fluids. We get about 20 percent of our water from food, so that amount needs to be replaced when fasting. Plus, as your body burns glycogen, it releases the water attached to it into your bloodstream and your kidneys expel it. You're releasing a lot more water than you're taking in. Without adequate water, you can't flush out all the toxins your body is excreting through burning up fat (a lot of toxins build up in fat) and the recycling process

TOP TACTIC

KEEP YOUR HANDS AND MIND BUSY

The number-one way to short-circuit a fast is to become preoccupied by any hunger you may feel. Keep your mind focused elsewhere. Answer emails, dig into a big assignment. Keep your hands busy, too. Tackle a home-improvement project, clean out your closets, romp with your kids. The busier you are, the less time you'll have to think about food and the less likely you'll be to break your fast ahead of schedule by eating out of boredom.

of autophagy. You can see why hydration becomes more important during a fast.

There's also a metabolic benefit to drinking water. Researchers have found that chugging 2¼ cups (600 ml) of water increased metabolism by 30 percent for 30 to 40 minutes. It shocks the body, increasing epinephrine levels. Now, we don't want to chug to the point where we harm ourselves, but drinking adequate amounts of water will keep your metabolism elevated.[46]

Odds are, you'll want to consume something during your fast, so staying hydrated should come easily. Keep it simple. When in doubt, drink plain water, coffee, and tea and drink more of it than you normally would.

→ **Making a fast harder with a stressed out mind-set.** Mind-set makes or breaks a fast. If you're stressed out, you won't be able to sustain the fast, let alone make it a sustainable lifestyle. Intermittent fasting stresses the body already—and that's what elicits the positive physical response we want—but we don't need to let that shake us mentally. Meditation, a nap, a walk, or other relaxation techniques are all ways to lower stress, anxiety, and monkey mind. A quick mindfulness session once or twice a day using an app such as Headspace will make fasting easier. Find a practice that works for you and make it a regular part of your fasting routine, especially during the last third of your fast to prevent cortisol from spiking before breaking the fast. Even better, make this type of self-care part of your everyday routine.

CHECKLIST

THE FASTING WINDOW MADE EASY

You won't go wrong if you follow these ten essential tips during your fasting window.

- ☐ Aim to fast for a minimum of twelve hours.
- ☐ Fast every other day, or less frequently.
- ☐ Eat a pre-fast meal that is high in fat and low in carbs.
- ☐ Stay hydrated with plenty of plain water, coffee, and tea (preferably green tea).
- ☐ Supplement with sodium, potassium, and magnesium to balance electrolytes.
- ☐ Save sweeteners, creamers, and other supplements for after the fast.
- ☐ Use dried spices, such as ginger and cayenne pepper, to deepen your fast, add flavor to beverages, and handle hunger.
- ☐ Promote a relaxed mind-set.
- ☐ Work out.
- ☐ Do what helps you achieve the results you're after and makes you feel good.

A sniff of dark chocolate can suppress appetite. Sounds wild, right? I thought so, too, but researchers have reported that smelling 85 percent cacao chocolate decreased levels of the hunger hormone ghrelin.[47] Full disclosure: I tried it and it killed my appetite for, maybe, fifteen minutes, and then I just wanted to eat the chocolate. My point? This tactic doesn't work for me, but it could work for you, like it has for others.

TROUBLESHOOTING

Set yourself up for success by knowing what to expect and being ready to problem solve some common issues that crop up during the fasting window. These issues are completely manageable, so don't let the side effects or challenges shift your focus from all the good stuff. I'm here to tell you that you can deal with anything that comes up, and if you stick with intermittent fasting, you can have success with it.

How should I handle hunger?

Hunger will hurt your adherence to the fast, so we need to find ways to combat these hunger pangs. Women are more sensitive to the hunger hormones leptin and ghrelin, so you may be hungrier at the start of a fast. Make sure you're getting adequate vitamins and minerals before you start your fast, which will prevent your body from sending the type of deficiency signals to the brain that can lead to hunger. If you're still getting the growlies, here are a few things to try.

→ **Add fenugreek to your pre-fast meal.** This herb, native to the Mediterranean region, contains galactomannan fiber, which holds exponentially more water than a typical soluble fiber.[48] Eating raw fenugreek seed powder with your pre-fast meal will draw water into your small intestine, causing the fiber to swell and keep you satiated for a good amount of time without preventing you from getting into a fasted state. Interestingly,

one study has shown that fenugreek seed extract also causes a big increase in satiety, even though it doesn't contain galactomannan fiber.[49] Researchers aren't yet sure why, but it could be worth a try given the positive effect it's been shown to have.

→ **Add shirataki noodles to your pre-fast meal.** Rich in glucomannan fiber, shirataki noodles will keep you satiated. Like galactomannan fiber, glucomannan fiber absorbs water and takes up space in your stomach and intestines for a long time, making you feel full. It can inhibit the absorption of certain minerals such as calcium, so be sure to support your body with a well-rounded variety of vitamins and minerals.[50]

Galactomannan and glucomannan fibers aren't magic bullets; they will make you feel full at the start of a fast but won't kill a desire for food. And, although they won't delay the onset of a fasted state, they will delay gut restoration. Your gut needs to be empty to reset, so if your main reason for fasting is digestive recovery, you may want to reconsider this strategy.

→ **Leverage cayenne pepper, ginger, green tea, and yerba mate.** Upregulating how much fat the body uses from our tissues can kill our hunger response. If it's getting enough fat, getting enough "to eat," your body is satiated, and you should feel less hungry. Drink green tea and yerba mate, or add ginger to your beverages, to feel more satisfied.[51] Or, kick your stress response into gear and dampen your hunger with a dash of cayenne pepper.[52] The shock of the spice reduces appetite but may cause tummy troubles, so avoid this if you have a sensitive stomach.

What do I do if I experience _____ during my fast?

→ **Headache.** A nagging low-grade ache over your forehead is a typical "fasting headache" caused by small changes in blood glucose altering the pain receptors in your brain a bit so you feel pain that isn't really there.[53] Dehydration and low salt could be factors with headache, though, so drink plenty of fluids and electrolytes. Added stress is also a factor. Surges of cortisol cause blood pressure to increase and put pressure on the nerve endings in your brain. Promoting a relaxed mind-set will help, and over time, as your body adapts to fasting, the headaches usually go away.

This type of headache is not the result of low blood sugar, or hypoglycemia. Blood glucose only decreases a bit while fasting as cells become more insulin sensitive and shift from running on glucose to running on fat. The liver steps up to create glucose through gluconeogenesis to keep the brain and other cells that rely on glucose fully stocked. Now, I'm not saying low blood sugar can't happen, but it is uncommon. Each individual is different. If you feel an incessant boom-boom throbbing headache, it may be a sign of low blood sugar and you might need to break your fast a bit earlier until your body adjusts.

→ **Diarrhea.** Not uncommon. It's usually caused by an improvement of gut motility and food moving through your system more quickly. It should resolve on its own.

→ **Brain fog and low energy.** Make sure you're well-hydrated and getting enough electrolytes. You could also try supplementing with 0.5 to 2 grams of creatine. It won't break your fast and it gives your brain a boost by creating more ATP, the main energy-carrying molecule in the body. Creatine works best when it has a chance to build up over time, rather than as an immediate fix when you're feeling a slump. Replenish your creatine stores by supplementing regularly to feel the most benefit.[54]

Why do I get so cold while fasting?

Grab an extra sweater because you're burning fat. As subcutaneous fat changes into visceral fat and burns, we lose some of the metabolically active brown fat that generates heat. To be clear: You're not getting cold because your metabolism is slowing. It's quite the opposite; your metabolism is speeding up. Drinking hot coffee is one way to warm yourself, and the caffeine stimulates orexin, a neurotransmitter associated with body temperature that when elevated will mitigate the cold you feel from fasting.[55]

Why is my sleep messed up?

Sleeplessness is a common issue and is usually the result of beginning or breaking your fasting window late in the day and, therefore, eating late at night, say at 8, 9, or 10 p.m. Eating so late disrupts your circadian rhythm and dysregulates the release of melatonin, the sleep-promoting hormone. Adjust your fasting window so you eat earlier in the day and avoid eating past dark.

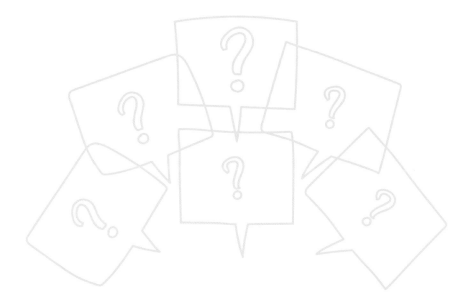

LET'S BREAK IT DOWN

- Eat a modest pre-fast meal that is high in fat and as low in carbs as possible with an apple cider vinegar "lemonade" (see page 68) to help get you into a fasted state quickly.

- Most foods and drinks with a caloric value, and/or an ingredient that raises insulin, will kick you out of a fasted state. Keep it simple with plain water, coffee, and tea (especially green tea).

- Replenish your electrolytes (sodium, potassium, and magnesium) during your fasting window and save other vitamins and supplements for afterward.

- Use cayenne pepper, cinnamon, ginger, and turmeric to help get more out of your fast. The benefits far outweigh the few calories consumed.

- Work out during your fasting window, especially with strength training. Keep it light or at the level where your body can easily recover.

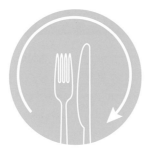

CHAPTER 5

Breaking Your Fast

The success of your fast is determined by how you break it. That's right. Breaking your fast is probably more important than the actual fast itself. So, it's imperative to break your fast properly. Always. By the end of your fasting window, your body is very sensitive, so you want to make sure you're only taking in the right stuff.

It's inevitable: Breaking your fast causes inflammation.[1] That's just the way it goes. You're at a crossroads. You can control the inflammation, or you can eat foods that trigger more inflammation. I think you know which path to take. Here's what the road ahead involves:

→ **Controlling insulin.** We always want to be in control of insulin. Everything we eat—carbs, fats, proteins—causes an insulin spike. Sometimes, a spike can be a good thing, as when we are trying to build muscle—but the key word is "control."

→ **Controlling cortisol.** If our cortisol levels are high when we break our fast, we risk accumulating fat, especially around the belly.

→ **Going easy on the gut.** At the end of a fast, our guts are fragile. Fasting temporarily weakens the intestinal mucosal barrier, the cell lining that acts as a selective barrier protecting you from bacteria, toxins, and undigested food escaping the gut and leaching into your bloodstream.[2] Irritating the gut can break down the gut wall, triggering inflammation and sparking a massive immune system response, which is the last thing you want to do. That's why, when breaking a fast, we want to avoid foods that can trigger inflammation, such as dairy and gluten, and eat anti-inflammatory foods that combat it.

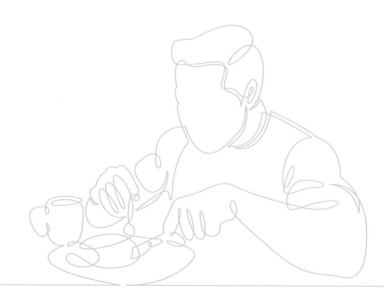

WHAT TO EAT AND DRINK *BEFORE* YOU BREAK YOUR FAST

Before we get to what you should eat to break your fast, we need to step back to about thirty minutes before your fasting window closes. Why? To make sure we suppress our cortisol levels so they aren't elevated when you do break your fast.

Because cortisol is associated with stress, you might think of it as a "bad" hormone, but it's actually quite good for us during a fast and helps with fat burning.[3] But, when high cortisol is combined with high insulin, it causes the opposite to happen: fat storage, especially around the middle.

Now, we can't fast indefinitely. We do have to eat, and when we do, our insulin will rise naturally. We can blunt the impact of increased insulin by keeping cortisol levels in check before we break our fast. Relaxation techniques, such as meditation, deep breathing exercises, or a walk outside, will help lower stress levels, but alone, they likely won't lower them enough because you're fasting and already physiologically stressed. Here's what I suggest you do about thirty minutes before breaking your fast:

→ **Add a dash of ground cinnamon** to your water, herbal tea, or decaf coffee. Cinnamon acts like insulin in the body, triggering cells to open and let the excess glucose in our bloodstream inside. By driving down your blood glucose levels, you drive your cortisol levels a little bit lower, too.

→ **Consume extra salt.** Sprinkling an additional bit of salt on your beverages (remember, while fasting you should add salt to any approved beverages you consume) will help keep you minerally balanced and lower cortisol. Here's how: Cortisol has a direct relationship with salt. Low sodium levels (which could happen after a longer fast) are correlated with increased cortisol levels.[4] If we increase our sodium with an extra sprinkle of salt, our body backs off producing aldosterone, the main hormone regulating salt and water in the body. Slowing aldosterone pushes cortisol levels down.[5]

→ **Supplement with magnesium.** After fasting, you can expect to be depleted of magnesium, shown to drive up cortisol levels.[6] Take a few magnesium tablets to bring the cortisol levels back down. Magnesium works by calming your nervous system, restricting the release of cortisol, and acting as a filter to prevent it from entering the brain.

By tag-teaming a little cinnamon with a little extra salt with a little magnesium, you'll lower insulin and cortisol levels and be in a better place to break your fast. This is especially important if you work out toward the end of your fast as your cortisol will be high.

BREAKING YOUR FAST: WHAT TO EAT AND AVOID

Your cells are going to absorb whatever you put into your body immediately after your fast like a sponge, so be very careful. When breaking your fast, eat a very controlled diet. The good news: just for this one meal. The rest of the day you have a lot more flexibility. Once you find a few favorite foods, you'll find breaking a fast easy. Let's start with the cardinal rules for *everyone*, no matter what eating style you follow.

→ **Eat a mini break-fast meal first, followed by a normal-size meal sixty to ninety minutes later.** It's best to break your fast with a small or mini break-fast meal first. Just a tiny portion of food lets your digestive system restart gently. Breaking your fast with a mini meal allows you to maintain control of the insulin spike that accompanies the consumption of any food (carbs, fats, proteins) and prevents you from inadvertently going overboard with a big meal. Sixty to ninety minutes after your mini meal, you can have a normal meal following your usual eating style, and then you can eat as you like for the rest of your eating window.

For your mini break-fast meal:
→ **Keep it lean.** Always break your fast with some lean protein: lean grass-fed, grass-finished chicken, pork, or turkey (though, turkey is not the best option as it's usually high in antibiotics) or high-quality wild sockeye salmon or white fish (cod, halibut, sea bass). Lean protein causes more moderate insulin and cortisol spikes than carbs and fats do.[7] We still want to keep both of these substances in check. Grass-finished meats, particularly beef, contain more omega-3 fatty acids than grain-fed meats, which break down quickly and easily and suppress the amount of lipopolysaccharide (LPS), a highly inflammatory agent, in the bloodstream.[8]

Protein also helps our mitochondria return to full energy production. Although fasting increases our mitochondrial efficiency, studies have demonstrated that it decreases the activity of the mitochondrial protein complexes, essential for energy production. Protein bounces those mitochondria back in a way carbs don't.[9] And, lean protein is a great way to replenish phosphorus and thiamine (vitamin B_1), both of which become depleted while fasting. We need phosphorus for energy production whereas thiamine supports fat and glucose metabolism.[10]

Stay away from red meat because it's higher in saturated fats, which are harder to break down at the end of a fast and have been linked to increased amounts of LPS.[11] Also, avoid shellfish as it contains thiaminase, an enzyme that prevents us from utilizing thiamine properly. At the end of our fast, we're pretty darn depleted of thiamine already, and breaking the fast with shellfish would make us more deficient.

What does lean protein mean for a vegan or vegetarian? Hemp or pea protein powder (no artificial sweeteners), sacha inchi, nutritional yeast, and teff, a gluten-free whole grain high in protein. Avoid whey protein powder because it's made from dairy.

→ **Do not mix fats and carbohydrates.** That means no combining a rice cake with almond butter or a greasy steak with a piece of bread. The reasoning is simple: Carbs cause an insulin spike that opens the cell doors for the carbs (in the form of glucose) *and* the fat to enter. More fat in our cells is exactly what we want to avoid.

Plus, fat raises levels of acylation stimulating hormone (ASP), which increases insulin.[12] When you consume fat with carbs, you get a bigger insulin spike than if you just had carbs. Disclaimer: Some fats slow the digestion of carbs and limit the severity of the insulin spike, but let's keep it simple:

When breaking your fast,

FATS + CARBS = NO!

Feel free to combine fats and carbs later in your eating window, but definitely do not combine them when you break a fast.

→ **No dairy (A1 and A2).** When A1 milk (the most common type of cow's milk) is digested, it produces beta-casomorphin 7 (BCM7).[13] This peptide is hard to break down and highly inflammatory, associated with abdominal pain, bloating, and gas, and, over time, a shortening of the intestinal villi, compromising the gut's ability to absorb nutrients.[14] BCM7 is best

TOP TACTIC

BREAK YOUR FAST WITH LEAN PROTEIN *ONLY*

Stop right here: All you need to break your fast is lean protein. That's it. I know it's boring. I know it's bland. But, if you want to make breaking your fast ridiculously easy, stick to lean protein only for your mini breakfast meal. Have a piece of lean poultry, pork, or fish, a protein powder shake (made with water), or some teff, and you won't go wrong. Keep it interesting by switching it up. For my favorite sources of lean protein, check out FastingIsEasy.com.

avoided, period, but certainly when your gut is known to be sensitive. A2 milk doesn't cause the same inflammatory response as A1 milk (the protein it contains does not produce BCM7) and has even been shown to improve gut villi in mice, but its high saturated-fat content makes it a poor choice with which to break a fast.[15]

→ **No beans.** Beans are high in lectins, a type of protein humans can't digest. Their traveling through your intestines unchanged causes irritation and damage. Lectins have also been dubbed an antinutrient because they can interfere with the absorption of calcium, iron, phosphorus, and zinc.[16] After a fast, it's essential to *promote* mineral absorption, so skip the beans.

→ **No veggies.** Don't get me wrong—I'm a big proponent of consuming lots and lots of veggies because of their tremendous health benefits. But, breaking a fast is not the time to load up. Because your gut is fragile, any food you eat to break your fast may stay in the stomach and small intestine longer than usual, increasing your risk of experiencing small bacterial intestinal overgrowth (SIBO), or too many bacteria in your small intestine. Veggies increase this likelihood because they contain certain sugars, such as raffinose, that are hard to digest and skew bacteria growth in a not-so-good way. Consuming the insoluble fiber found in vegetables such as Brussels sprouts, carrots, celery, kale, and leafy greens is like shoving a wire brush against your fragile intestinal villi, making it harder to absorb nutrients. Say no to vegetables for your mini break-fast meal and ease up on your digestion.

→ **No nuts.** The phytic acid and oxalates in nuts inhibit the absorption of minerals such as calcium, iron, magnesium, and zinc—all of which we want and need after a fast.[17] "No nuts" includes almond, cashew, and other nut milks. Use water, hemp, flax, or coconut milk to make a protein shake.

→ **No soy.** I know this can be hard if you are vegan or vegetarian, but after a day of fasting don't turn to soy, which contains phytic acid, dubbed an "antinutrient" because it binds to vital minerals (calcium, iron, magnesium, and zinc) and vitamins (A, B_{12}, D, and E), making them less available to our bodies.[18]

→ **No gluten.** Gluten, a protein contained in many grains, including barley, rye, and wheat, is highly inflammatory for many people and best avoided when breaking a fast. Avoiding gluten is key for women because of the role it may play when it comes to thyroid health. Gluten contains gliadin, a protein with two potentially damaging qualities: 1) It triggers the release of zonulin, which loosens the tight junctions of the intestinal mucosal barrier; and 2) the antibodies to gliadin are similar in molecular structure to thyroid antibodies.[19] If gliadin enters the bloodstream through a weak intestinal mucosal barrier, the body attacks it as a foreign invader *and* may attack the thyroid, too. Don't risk it.

To keep it extra easy on your body on a fasting day, consider eliminating grains entirely, as even corn, quinoa, rice, and other grains contain agglutinin, a type of protein that is difficult to digest and linked to an inflammatory immune system response.[20]

→ **Do drink green tea.** Green tea is excellent for gut support, capable of restoring the intestinal villi that atrophy during a fast and improving the integrity of the gut lining and fighting inflammation.[21]

Follow these cardinal rules and you will be well on your way to successfully breaking your fast, but if you want to get a little more nuanced and do more to support your body based on your preferred eating style, use the following recommendations for your mini break-fast meal and beyond.

BREAKING YOUR FAST BASICS

1. Eat a mini break-fast meal.

2. Sixty to ninety minutes later, eat a normal-size meal following your usual eating style.

FOR YOUR MINI BREAK-FAST MEAL

Eat	Avoid
✓ Green tea	✗ Beans
✓ Lean protein	✗ Dairy
	✗ Gluten
	✗ Mixing fats and carbohydrates
	✗ Nuts
	✗ Soy
	✗ Veggies

Keto: Mini Break-Fast Meal

The goal is to extend the life of the fast as long as possible and break your fast with lean proteins and healthy fats that will allow you to produce the most ketones.

EAT

✅ **LEAN PROTEIN** (3 to 6 ounces, or 85 to 170 g) or a lean protein shake made with pea or hemp protein. If you are over age forty, I recommend using this calculation to determine how much protein to use to break your fast: Take your weight in pounds, find 25 percent of it, and prepare that many grams of lean protein. So, if you weigh 200 pounds (91 kg), you would eat 50 grams (1¾ ounces) of protein.

✅ **BONE BROTH** (3 to 4 ounces, or 90 to 120 ml). The gelatin in bone broth draws water into your intestinal tract, protecting the gut mucosal layer to help you utilize more of the nutrients you're consuming without gut distress. Collagen is broken down into amino acids such as glycine and proline, the building blocks for new collagen, to help restore the gut long term. Bone broth also contains glutamine, vital for gut lining integrity, and a lot of minerals to restore what's been lost while fasting.[22]

✅ **A COUPLE CAPSULES OF OMEGA-3 FATTY ACID SUPPLEMENTS.** It's hard to get enough omega-3s during a fasting day through food alone. Omega-3s aid the absorption of protein, helping preserve and build muscle and control the post-fast-breaking inflammatory response by lowering LPS levels, which is phenomenally good news.[23] I like algal or calamarine oil (derived from squid or calamari) because the lower you go down the food chain, the more potent the omega-3s are.

✅ **APPLE CIDER VINEGAR.** The acetic acid in apple cider vinegar helps bring down blood sugar so we avoid a wild spike coming out of the fast, and it supports the microbiome by breaking down biofilms, colonies of bad bacteria.[24]

✅ **SEAWEED (IODINE), FOR WOMEN.** Have some seaweed snacks or flavor lean protein with seaweed flakes to replenish your iodine stores, an essential mineral for the production of thyroid hormone. The thyroid combines iodine and the amino acid tyrosine to make triiodothyronine (T3) and thyroxine (T4), the active and inactive forms of thyroid hormone.[25] Your body doesn't make iodine, so you have to get it from outside sources. Thyroid health is especially important for women and, after fasting, we want to give the thyroid all the support it needs.

AVOID

❌ **FATS.** Goes against the grain, right? You're keto and you want to break that fast with fat. For this one meal, you need to control it—no extra fat beyond what's already in the lean protein, bone broth, and omega-3 supplement.

❌ **CARBS.** Keep it low carb.

Keto: Normal-Size Meal (Sixty to Ninety Minutes Later)

This meal is all about renourishing while remaining in a ketogenic state to continue the fat burning and other benefits of the fast. You've already done a tremendous job increasing the production of ketones and, depending on the length of your fast, getting into ketosis during your fast, so, why not eat things that allow you to ride this wave for the rest of that day? Go to town on the right kind of fats and keep it low carb.

EAT

✔ **PROTEIN.** Enjoy those fattier cuts of meat now. You want omega-3s, so lean on Atlantic salmon, mackerel, and my personal favorite: sardines or grass-fed, grass-finished beef.

✔ **FATS.** Some types of fats are better than others.

> **(+) Polyunsaturated fats.** These healthy fats, rich in omega-3 fatty acids, break down quickly and easily and have been shown to generate significantly higher ketone levels when compared to saturated fats.[26]

> **(+) Fats rich in oleic acid.** Linked to lowering inflammation and mobilizing fat, oleic acid is found in olive oil and avocado oil (to a much lesser degree).[27]

> **(+) Fats rich in oleanolic acid.** Abundant in olive oil, oleanolic acid had been shown to block the breakdown of the gut.[28]

> **(-) MCTs.** These fats are rapidly absorbed but can cause the kind of gut distress that can really throw a wrench in your day.

> **(-) Saturated fats.** This type of fat is necessary for optimal brain and nerve health, but it's a good idea to limit saturated fat because it can trigger an increase in LPS into the bloodstream.[29] Saturated fat also takes a longer time to break down, which can stress the gut.

✔ **CRUCIFEROUS VEGGIES.** I'm a fan of Brussels sprouts, but all cruciferous vegetables are high in indole-3-carbinol, which our bodies metabolize into diindolylmethane (DIM). DIM promotes a healthy hormone balance of estrogen in both men and women.[30] And the sulforaphane in these vegetables reduces inflammation. I like having some deep green with this meal and these vegetables are solid choices.

✔ **SOLUBLE FIBER.** The soluble fiber found in chia and flax is fuel for your gut. It degrades into short chain fatty acids that heal the gut and signal the brain to utilize fats more efficiently.[31]

PREBIOTIC-RICH FOODS. You have more good bacteria at the end of a fast, so now is the time to light a fire and feed them with artichoke, asparagus, bok choy, cabbage, garlic, onion, and other prebiotic-rich veggies or resistant starches, such as chickpea and lentil flours or cooked, cooled, and re-heated potato or white rice. The cooking and cooling forms more resistant starch and lowers the glycemic load, or impact, that a serving of food has on blood sugar.

SHELLFISH, FOR WOMEN. Choose scallops, shrimp, or other types of shellfish to get protein with less connective tissue, so it absorbs better, plus copper iodine, selenium, and zinc to support your thyroid further.

AVOID

CARBS. We are still keeping it low carb.

Keto: Mini-Meal Before Bed (Optional)

If you break your fast late in the day and, after dinner, you're still a little hungry before bed, opt for some unsweetened Greek or Bulgarian yogurt with a tablespoon or two (16 to 32 g) of macadamia nut butter. It's okay to introduce a little dairy and a modest amount of nuts now, but keep the amount to a minimum and try to avoid nuts high in phytic acid, such as almonds, Brazil nuts, cashews, and hazelnuts. Go with macadamia nuts, pecans, or walnuts instead.

Consider adding coconut oil for the MCTs to help you sleep. MCTs have been shown to allow more tryptophan into the brain.[32] More tryptophan means more serotonin production, and more serotonin means more melatonin production. Melatonin lets your body know it's time to go to sleep.

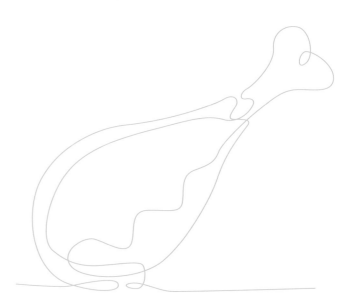

Non-Keto (Fasting with Carbs): Mini Break-Fast Meal

When fasting with carbs, it's critical to stay ultra-strict about separating fats and carbs. Eating them together will simply store all that fat, basically undoing all the work of your fast. Instead, for your mini meal, focus on carbs plus protein to shuttle all the protein into your cells and promote muscle preservation and growth. Save fats for a later meal.

EAT

✓ **LEAN PROTEIN** (3 to 6 ounces, or 85 to 170 g) or a lean protein shake made with pea or hemp protein. If you are over age forty, I recommend using this calculation to determine how much protein to use to break your fast: Take your weight in pounds, find 25 percent of it, and prepare that many grams of lean protein. So, if you weigh 200 pounds (91 kg), you would eat 50 grams (1¾ ounces) of protein.

✓ **A HIGH GLYCEMIC-LOAD CARB,** such as organic rice cakes or puffed rice cereal (no sugar added) or a plain baked white potato. If you eat carbs, you want a controlled insulin spike to end your fasting period and click off autophagy and click on mTOR.[33] It may sound a little nuts, but eating a high glycemic-load carb now, the type of carb that will release glucose into the bloodstream quickly, allowing a little dip, and then having a low glycemic-load carb sixty to ninety minutes later with your normal-size meal, will limit the spike. If you ate

HYDRATE! ESPECIALLY IF YOU ARE BREAKING YOUR FAST WITH CARBS

When you break your fast and your insulin levels rise, electrolytes get sucked out of the bloodstream and into cells, leaving you open to dehydration.[34] Carbs have a greater impact on insulin, so if you follow a non-keto eating plan, drink plenty of water with your mini break-fast meal.

a low glycemic-load carb with your mini break-fast meal, your insulin would still be at its peak for your normal-size meal. Adding more carbs on top of what you already ate leads to the type of sky-high levels we don't want to see.

Eating a carb with a lean protein will help move that protein into cells and encourage muscle growth and recovery. This strategy also helps restore muscle glycogen stores. Keep the portion size small; avoid going over 25 grams (scant 1 ounce).

✓ **A SMALL AMOUNT OF FRUCTOSE,** such as half a small orange or nectarine or a few berries. Fructose is a simple sugar found in fruits that doesn't trigger an insulin response. Combined with the high glycemic-load carb, it enhances the absorption of the carbs.

✅ **ANTIOXIDANTS,** such as a vitamin C supplement. Oxidative stress breaks down collagen, which is essential for healing and sealing the gut. Add antioxidants to support the collagen you already have and stimulate collagen production.[35]

✅ **A COUPLE CAPSULES OF OMEGA-3 FATTY ACIDS.** It's hard to get enough omega-3s during a fasting day through food alone. Omega-3s aid the absorption of protein, helping preserve and build muscle, and control the post-fast-breaking inflammatory response by lowering LPS levels, which is phenomenally good news for us.[36] I like algal or calamarine oil (derived from squid or calamari) because the lower you go down the food chain, the more potent the omega-3s.

✅ **APPLE CIDER VINEGAR.** The acetic acid in apple cider vinegar helps bring our blood sugar down so we avoid a wild spike coming out of the fast, and it supports the microbiome by breaking down biofilms, colonies of bad bacteria.[37]

✅ **SEAWEED (IODINE), FOR WOMEN.** Have some seaweed snacks or flavor lean protein with seaweed flakes to replenish your iodine stores, a mineral essential for the production of thyroid hormone. The thyroid combines iodine and the amino acid tyrosine to make triiodothyronine (T3) and thyroxine (T4), the active and inactive forms of thyroid hormone. Your body doesn't make iodine, so you have to get it from outside sources. Thyroid health is especially important for women and, after fasting, we want to give the thyroid all the support it needs.

✅ **(ALTERNATIVE) BONE BROTH** (3 to 4 ounces, or 90 to 120 ml). Bone broth is high in fat, so only add it to your mini break-fast meal if you are skipping the high glycemic-load carbs and fructose. Bone broth does have some unique and potent benefits. The gelatin in bone broth draws water into your intestinal tract, protecting the gut mucosal layer to help you utilize more of the nutrients you're consuming without gut distress. Collagen is broken down into amino acids, such as glycine and proline, the building blocks for new collagen, to help restore the gut long term. Bone broth also contains glutamine, which is vital for gut lining integrity, and a lot of minerals to restore what's been lost during the fast.[38] Because you'll restore collagen with this broth, there is no need for the antioxidant supplement.

AVOID

❌ **FATS.** Keep fats out of the equation, except for the fat in the lean protein, omega-3 supplement, and bone broth.

TOP TACTIC

6 FOODS TO BREAK YOUR FAST ON THE GO

1. **Protein powder.** Put some hemp or pea protein in a baggie or to-go cup, mix with water: done.
2. **Pork, turkey, or venison jerky or sticks.** I almost always have these in my backpack.
3. **Smoked sockeye salmon.** A good grab-and-go option. To counteract the high sodium and avoid bloat city, take some magnesium.
4. **Lean, clean deli meat.** Admittedly, this can be tough to come by as most deli meat is chock-full of additives, antibiotics, flavorings, and pesticides! Your gut will thank you by keeping it to just a few slices and adding some magnesium to balance the high sodium.
5. **Hard-boiled egg white.** Yep, ditch the yolk to avoid the saturated fat. Eggs can be inflammatory for some people, so they aren't at the top of my list, but eggs may work just fine for you—on occasion.
6. **Unsweetened low-fat Greek or Bulgarian yogurt.** Not a top choice because I think it's best to stay away from dairy for your mini break-fast meal but, once in a while, in a pinch, it's not the worst way to go. The probiotics support the gut.

Non-Keto (Fasting with Carbs): Normal-Size Meal (Sixty to Ninety Minutes Later)

Add a more diverse array of foods to restock essential nutrients and focus on low glycemic-load carb while staying lean on protein.

EAT

✔ **PROTEIN.** Stick with leaner cuts of protein.

✔ **LOW GLYCEMIC LOAD—CARBOHYDRATES.** Control the second-wave insulin spike with acorn and butternut squash, beets, chana dal (a type of chickpea), chickpea pasta, lentils, parsnips, and split peas.

✔ **CRUCIFEROUS VEGGIES.** I'm a fan of Brussels sprouts, but all cruciferous vegetables are high in indole-3-carbinol, which our bodies metabolize into diindolylmethane (DIM).

DIM promotes a healthy hormone balance of estrogen in both men and women—and the sulforaphane reduces inflammation. I like having some deep greens with this meal and these vegetables are solid choices.

✅ **SOLUBLE FIBER.** The soluble fiber found in chia and flax is fuel for your gut. It degrades into short chain fatty acids that heal the gut and signal the brain to utilize fats better.[39]

✅ **PREBIOTIC-RICH FOODS.** Your gut has more good bacteria at the end of a fast, so now is the time to light a fire and feed them with artichokes, asparagus, bok choy, cabbage, garlic, onion, and other prebiotic-rich veggies or resistant starches, such as chickpea and lentil flours or cooked, cooled, and re-heated potatoes or white rice. (The cooking and cooling forms more resistant starch and lowers the glycemic load, or impact, a serving of a food has on blood sugar.)

✅ **SHELLFISH, FOR WOMEN.** Choose shrimp, scallops, or other types of shellfish to get a lean protein with less connective tissue, so it absorbs better, plus copper, iodine, selenium, and zinc to further support your thyroid.

AVOID

❌ **FATS.** Keep additional fat off the plate for now.

Non-Keto (Fasting with Carbs): Mini-Meal

For those consuming carbs, I recommend another mini-meal a few hours after your normal-size meal to get some fats in your system.

EAT

✅ **FAT.** Choose unsweetened Greek or Bulgarian yogurt with a tablespoon or two (16 to 32 g) of macadamia nut butter. It's okay to introduce a little dairy and a modest amount of nuts now, but keep the amount to a minimum, and try to avoid nuts high in phytic acid, such as almonds, Brazil nuts, cashews, and hazelnuts. Go with macadamia nuts, pecans, or walnuts instead.

If this mini meal lands close to your bedtime, consider adding coconut oil for the MCTs to help you sleep. MCTs have been shown to allow more tryptophan into the brain.[40] More tryptophan means more serotonin production, and more serotonin means more melatonin production. Melatonin lets your body know it's time to go to sleep.

AVOID

❌ **CARBS.** Because you're amping up the fats, keep the carbs low.

Vegans and vegetarians can follow the preceding recommendations noted for a keto or a non-keto eating plan and make these substitutions and additions.

Vegan and Vegetarian: Mini Break-Fast Meal

EAT

✓ **A COUPLE CAPSULES OF ALGAE OIL/ALGAE DHA.** A vegan- and vegetarian-friendly source of the omega-3 fatty acids. It's hard to get enough omega-3s during a fasting day through food alone. Vegans and vegetarians tend to be low in omega-3s anyway, so I suggest supplementing to keep these levels up and inflammation at bay.[41] Omega-3s aid the absorption of protein, helping preserve and build muscle, and control the post-fast-breaking inflammatory response by lowering LPS levels, which is phenomenally good news for us.[42]

Vegan and Vegetarian: Normal-Size Meal (Sixty to Ninety Minutes Later)

EAT

✓ **A COUPLE CAPSULES OF ALGAE OIL/ALGAE DHA.** I recommend supplementing with this for each meal during the eating window of your fasting day.

Vegan and Vegetarian: Mini-Meal Before Bed (Keto, Optional)/Mini Meal (Non-Keto)

EAT

✓ **A COUPLE CAPSULES OF ALGAE OIL/ALGAE DHA.**

✓ **UNSWEETENED COCONUT YOGURT.** Have this nondairy yogurt option with macadamia nut butter.

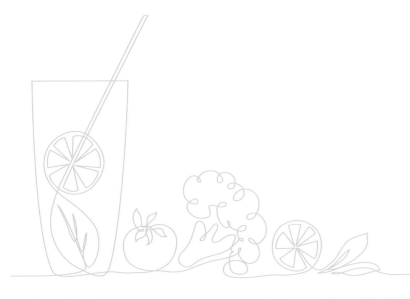

FAST BREAK PHO

Inspired by Vietnamese pho, this is a seriously good, simple, savory soup with which to break a fast.

Ingredients

- 1 carton (7 to 10 ounces, or 210 to 300 ml) high-quality bone broth (I alternate between chicken and beef)

- 5 ounces (140 g) superlean chicken or turkey

- Ground ginger

- Tamari (not soy sauce; it contains gluten)

- Handful of rice noodles (for non-keto eaters)

- 3 tablespoons (45 ml) apple cider vinegar

- Seaweed flakes

In a saucepan over medium-high heat, heat the bone broth until it is warmed through. Add the chicken or turkey. Season to taste with ginger (I add a couple teaspoons) and tamari. Simmer until the protein is nearly done. If you are not keto, add the rice noodles and cook until the noodles are tender. Pour in the vinegar and sprinkle with seaweed flakes. (Add both of these ingredients when the soup is just about ready to serve, so you don't denature the probiotics in the vinegar or break down too much of the phytonutrients in the seaweed.) Enjoy! You can cook this soup ahead and refrigerate for later use.

AVOID THESE COMMON MISTAKES

As you've learned, how you break your fast is a major factor in your results—maybe even *the* most important factor. To get the most benefit from your fast, avoid these hiccups.

→ **Not reducing cortisol levels before breaking your fast.** It's important to be careful about cortisol at the end of your fast because high cortisol levels can undo much of the good from the fast. Women are especially prone to high levels of cortisol. Take extra care to use cinnamon, magnesium, and salt in the last thirty minutes or so of your fast to reduce cortisol levels.

→ **Eating a big meal right away.** The tendency at the end of a fast is to raid the pantry and dive into a large meal comprising a variety of foods. I've been there. Unfortunately, this approach can backfire. At the end of your fast, you have a golden period where your whole body's insulin sensitivity is increased, meaning your cells are much more capable of absorbing nutrients.[43] This can be a very good thing, but some studies show that when you eat too much, your body perceives these excess nutrients as a threat and fights back, triggering an inflammatory response.

The abundance of nutrients consumed in one sitting is just too much for the cells to handle. Instead of processing those nutrients, your body resists absorbing them and responds by releasing protein kinase R (PKR), which points out and fights viruses.[44] This leads to a massive round of inflammation, defeating everything you're trying to do by fasting. That's why I recommend breaking your fast with a modest meal, followed by one, or even two, spaced-out meals. Break your fast in a controlled way with a little bit of lean protein and then get more flexible.

→ **Working out immediately after breaking your fast.** Of course, it's entirely up to you when you work out, but if you are looking to maximize the benefits of fasting and optimize

your results *a lot*, work out in a fasted state instead. Even better: Work out at the tail end of your fast when you'll burn the most fat. You may see some performance decline at that point, but you should still be able to work out hard and reap the effects of the fast, including more fat loss, better muscle building, and improved muscle recovery.

I know it can be frustrating not to be at 100 percent, but what matters is that your relative strength is improving. Compare apples to apples. If each time you work out in a fasted state, you see gains, then you're good. Working out should always be challenging; it's the only way to improve and develop that element of skill that makes you a better athlete and person.

If you decide to work out after you eat, give yourself some time to digest the food first. As soon as you break your fast, blood rushes to your stomach and digestive tract to help you digest the food. Working out immediately after eating takes that blood away from your vital organs and sends it to your extremities, compromising your ability to absorb nutrients. And anyway, why would you want to work out with a pile of undigested food sitting in your stomach, making you feel bloated and icky? Do yourself a favor—wait a little while after breaking your fast and then exercise.

TROUBLESHOOTING

Following are some of the most common questions I get about breaking a fast. Knowing how to handle these issues will help you achieve results faster, avoid plateaus, and stick with intermittent fasting.

I'm so hungry after I break my fast. How can I prevent overeating and erasing everything I've accomplished by fasting?

Prioritize protein.[45] Make sure you consume enough protein in your mini break-fast meal and in your normal-size meal sixty to ninety minutes later. It comes down to the protein leverage hypothesis, which states that because we do not have a way to store protein, we will eat until our protein needs have been met.[46] If we eat excess carbs, we can store them as muscle and liver glycogen and, ultimately, fat. If we overeat fat, we can store it as fat. If we overeat protein, we don't store it as protein. It gets converted to fat and surplus amino acids are excreted. So, it makes sense that the body prioritizes protein to make sure we get enough. Generally, we remain somewhat hungry until our protein needs are met.

If we've been fasting, of course our protein needs haven't been met. It doesn't really matter during the fasting window because the body is happily running on fats and in protein-protection mode. It's not exactly craving protein in the fasted state.

But, once a single calorie hits your tongue, it's a different world. What happens in the fed world is far different than in the fasting world.

It's eating time, and the body shifts gears to protein prioritization. Your body is craving protein, protein, protein, but you don't necessarily know this. All you feel is a flood of hunger hormones. What do we usually reach for when we're feeling insatiable? I'll give you a hint: not protein. You could eat 5,000 calories of carbs and fats and you'd probably still feel hungry because your protein needs have not been met. We need protein to satiate us.

The solution: Beat your body to the punch by getting adequate protein within the first few hours after your fast. Have protein with your mini break-fast meal and again with your normal-size meal sixty to ninety minutes later. How much protein? A standard guideline for protein requirements is 0.7 to 0.8 grams per pound of body weight. This varies widely depending on your body composition, how hard you work out, and so on. Don't get lost in the details. Lean on protein in the hours after you break your fast.

And with your normal-size meal, add some soluble fiber, such as chia and flax, to help with satiation. This indigestible fiber takes a while to make its way through your digestive tract, providing a feeling of fullness and prompting your body to release fewer hunger hormones. You'll make better choices when the hunger alarm bells aren't ringing.

SLOW DOWN

Eat *slowly*. Chew your food well before swallowing it. Researchers have found that chewing your food more thoroughly significantly aids digestion and results in better absorption of nutrients.[47] Chewing your food well also gives your body a chance to register satiety. In one small study, adults who increased the number of chews per bite from fifteen to forty ate fewer calories and had lower levels of ghrelin, a hunger hormone.

I feel great during my fasting window, but once I break my fast, I feel bloated and puffy. What can I do?

While fasting, the lining that protects our gut, the gut mucosal lining, weakens as part of the breakdown and regeneration process. That weakened lining means that, during the short window of time between ending your fast and eating, your gut is at its most vulnerable. Make sure you choose the right foods to break your fast and give your gut a chance to reset, which means avoiding inflammatory foods, such as dairy and gluten, and vegetables. Review the complete list beginning on page 94 or make it easy on yourself and choose protein alone to break your fast.

You may be sensitive to foods high in FODMAPs, a type of carbohydrate that isn't always completely digested or absorbed in the intestines and, so, results in bloating, gas, and general gut havoc. Easing up on high-FODMAP foods such as asparagus, Brussels sprouts, cauliflower, chickpeas, garlic, lentils, and onions in the hours immediately following the end of a fast could make a big difference in how you feel.[48]

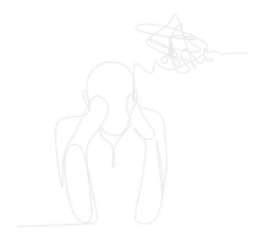

I have an energy slump after breaking my fast. What gives?

Your digestive system was on break during your fast, but once you eat something, it kicks back into gear, and that uses a lot of energy. Taking some proteolytic digestive enzymes, the kind that help you break down and absorb protein, when you break your fast (because you are breaking your fast with lean protein, right?), can take some of the strain off your gut, aid digestion, and, ultimately, improve energy.[49] I don't use these enzymes every time I fast, but I've found that they help when I throw them into the mix.

Supplementing with coenzyme Q10 immediately after breaking a fast will help boost energy by quickly restoring the activity of your mitochondrial complexes.[50] During the fast, you didn't feel like you had less energy because of the upregulation of those high-octane ketones. But, once you break your fast and stop producing ketones, you just might feel the difference because your mitochondria are still impaired. Breaking your fast with protein will help, but it may not be enough.

Adding a small amount of bee propolis, a resin-like compound bees make by combining their saliva and beeswax with oils, pollen, waxes, and other compounds from a tree's buds, sap, and flowers to your fast-breaking routine will reduce inflammation, which is another cause of post-fast sluggishness.[51] Bee propolis is also packed with B vitamins, including B_1 (thiamine), which gets depleted during a fast and needs to be restocked for efficient glucose metabolism. Without B_1, your body has to work harder to draw energy from any carbohydrates you may eat when breaking your fast, putting you in a slump.[52]

LET'S BREAK IT DOWN

- *How* you break your fast determines the success of your fast. It's that important. Break your fast properly. Always.

- Bring insulin and cortisol levels down before breaking your fast. About thirty minutes before your fasting window ends, have a little bit of cinnamon, magnesium, and some extra salt to set you up right.

- Keep it super simple: Break your fast with a mini break-fast meal of lean protein and green tea only.

- Sixty to ninety minutes after your mini break-fast meal, eat a normal-size meal following your chosen eating style.

- Prioritize protein after breaking your fast to prevent overeating and ease up on inflammatory foods to give your sensitive gut a chance to reset.

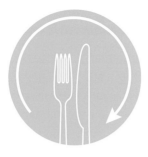

CHAPTER 6

Your Eating Window

I'm not here to convince you there's one right way to eat during your eating window (or on nonfasting days) or bash particular diets. But I want you to know how what you eat during your eating window and on nonfasting days affects the results you're trying to achieve with fasting—and your total health.

THE GOAL

To eat in a way that's best for your body, lifestyle, and health goals, the most important thing to do is to get adequate nutrients during your eating window. Making sure your body gets everything it needs is a good plan, in general, but it will also make intermittent fasting easier. Your body is unique and has a very powerful way of knowing when you are deficient in something and then telling your brain to eat so you get those needed vitamins and minerals. The best way to head off those hunger signals at the pass is to eat a well-rounded, nutrient-rich diet and supplement, as needed, to keep your body fully stocked.

One of the biggest advantages of intermittent fasting is that it works with *any* diet. That said, depending on your health and fitness goals and personal preferences, there are pros and cons to some of the most popular eating plans, such as keto, non-keto, vegan, and vegetarian. I'll share the benefits of each and specific ways to get the most from their unique nutritional profiles.

One eating style is not necessarily better than another, though some are better at achieving certain goals than others. After maximum fat loss? Go with keto. Focused on building muscle? Fasting with carbs has advantages. "Best" really depends on what you're after, and what you're after can change—so can your preferences. I eat mostly a keto diet, but sometimes I eat carbs, pescatarian, vegan, vegan keto—cycling in and out and always incorporating intermittent fasting. I like each for different reasons.

I'm not going to dive into the specifics of each plan. There are many excellent books and resources for that (visit FastingIsEasy.com for some suggestions). Instead, the focus here is on how each eating plan offers some unique opportunities and challenges when it comes to intermittent fasting.

Keto

The ketogenic diet of reducing carbs and eating higher amounts of fats uniquely complements intermittent fasting. The two work together harmoniously because they both rely on ketones.

One of the benefits of fasting is the creation of ketones during gluconeogenesis, and then, after enough time, switching to this high-octane fuel as the dominant source of energy. Ketones bring a lot of benefits: They are anti-inflammatory, promote the regeneration of gut stem cells, and are the most efficient brain fuel, being at the root of sharper thinking, focus, and memory.

The ketogenic diet is designed to get the body running on ketones, a process called ketosis, without fasting. Instead of not eating for a length a time initiating the creation of ketones, making certain dietary choices puts the body into that highly efficient fat-burning and ketone-producing state.

Intermittent fasting and the ketogenic diet share the same goal, to promote ketone production. They just approach it in two different ways.

One of the best ways a keto diet can leverage the benefits of intermittent fasting is by extending the benefits of your fast. If you stay strictly keto in your eating and don't have any carbs when you break your fast (or follow the recommendations in chapter 5), you'll stay in ketosis and a fasted state. Once you consume carbs, you kick your body out of ketosis and a fasted state and back into running on glucose for fuel. A keto diet along with fasting works really well to enhance the effects of

MOST NUTRIENT DEFICIENCIES
COME FROM TWO THINGS:

1. Eating the same foods over and
over again, without enough variety.

2. Depleted growing soil, which results
in plants with fewer vitamins and minerals.

It is important to make a concerted effort to eat a
balanced *and* diverse assortment of foods while
paying attention to where those foods come from.
Deficiencies are easy to fix if you pay attention.

each. You get more of the benefits of fasting, including accelerated fat loss, clearer thinking, and improved ability to manufacture energy, without having to extend your fasting window.

And, just quickly, to dispel one of the most persistent myths about keto—it is not just a bunch of dairy, meat, and other animal proteins. True keto relies on fats coming from healthy plant sources and limiting meat. Keto and plant-based work really well together.

Non-Keto

You will get the advantages of intermittent fasting while eating carbs but, full disclaimer, you won't lose as much fat or experience as much of a cognitive boost compared to following a keto diet. This difference results from jumping in and out of ketosis all the time instead of staying in it for extended periods. Just as your body starts to get used to utilizing body fat as fuel, you put carbs back into the equation and switch out of fat-burning mode.

Fasting with carbs does give you the chance to build a little more muscle because you can manipulate insulin spikes, especially effective when breaking your fast. Consuming carbs with protein to break your fast increases insulin and mTOR for muscle creation, while leveraging your insulin sensitivity to absorb a lot of that protein. That's all good for muscle growth.

To be strategic with your insulin spikes, you need to know that all carbs do not cause the same insulin response in the body. The glycemic load measures the impact one serving of food has on blood sugar.

High glycemic-load foods pass rapidly through your digestive system and into your bloodstream, driving up your blood glucose levels and causing insulin to spike. Obvious foods in this category include bagels, cornflakes, and pasta, but baked potatoes, raisins, and white rice fall into this category, too.

Low glycemic-load foods, on the other hand, pass through the digestive system more slowly and enter the bloodstream gradually, which keeps insulin levels low. These foods increase the body's sensitivity to insulin, keep you feeling fuller longer, and minimize energy crashes. Some of my favoriteLow glycemic-load foods include asparagus, bok choy, cabbage, lentils, spinach, and teff.

There are no "good" or "bad" carbs here, just carbs that influence your body in different ways. Understanding that difference will help you choose the right carbs at the right time and especially when breaking a fast.

Vegan and Vegetarian

It's more difficult, though not impossible, for vegans and vegetarians to get a sufficient and steady supply of all the essential minerals, nutrients, protein, and vitamins the body needs. When you fast, you add to that challenge by limiting potential nutritional opportunities because of the smaller eating window you create. So, vegans and vegetarians may need to plan and adjust their meals and supplements to make sure they consume a complete nutrient profile to thrive with intermittent fasting. If you're already vegan or vegetarian, you likely know what you need to eat to feel and function optimally. Intermittent fasting is an opportunity to refine your dietary approach. Three common deficiencies to watch out for are:[1]

→ Calcium
→ Omega-3s
→ Vitamin B$_{12}$

Ensuring you get enough protein is important for everyone but especially important if you're over age forty. During your eating window, it is beyond imperative that you get enough protein, and this will likely mean increasing the amount of protein at each meal to compensate for the lost meals while fasting. Aim to take in the same amount of protein you would usually consume over three meals on a nonfasting day in two meals on a fasting day. This is where a high-quality protein shake made with pea or hemp protein can help meet your needs.

Mediterranean Diet

Based on the traditional foods eaten by the people living in Mediterranean-area countries such as Italy and Greece, the Mediterranean diet is rich in plant-based foods, including fruit, herbs, legumes, nuts and seeds, olive oil, spices, vegetables, and whole grains with moderate amounts of dairy, fish, poultry, and seafood, and minimal consumption of red meat. Numerous studies have linked this diet to weight loss and a lower chance of developing chronic conditions.[2]

These foods not only align with intermittent fasting, but many of them also actively support it. Mediterranean spices, such as rosemary and oregano, have the capacity to switch on PPAR-alpha, the "key" to fasting, whereas olive oil, as a monounsaturated fat packed with oleic and oleanolic acid, lowers inflammation, mobilizes fat, and blocks the breakdown of the gut.

But what gets me really excited is, pairing a Mediterranean-style diet with intermittent fasting could be the ultimate way to reduce belly fat. Why? Both eating patterns have been shown to increase adiponectin, a hormone secreted by fat cells that helps us burn them up. By now, you may be tired of hearing about intermittent fasting incinerating fat, with CD36 pulling lipids into cells, turning white fat into heat-generating brown fat. These fat-burning mechanisms raise adiponectin. When it comes to the Mediterranean diet, high-quality monounsaturated fats, think olive oil, and omega-3s are key.

One study compared two groups:[3] One group consumed a diet made up of 65 percent carbohydrates, 6 percent saturated fat, 8 percent monounsaturated fat, and 6 percent polyunsaturated fats, such as omega-3s. The other group consumed 47 percent carbohydrates, 9 percent saturated fat, 23 percent monounsaturated fat coming largely from high-quality olive oil, and 6 percent polyunsaturated fats, again mainly from omega-3s. Both groups ate the same number of calories. The researchers found that the group on the

2MAD INSTEAD OF OMAD

I'm not a big fan of one meal a day (OMAD). Why?

- It forces you to stuff all your calories into one meal, which can overwhelm your body, prevent the absorption of nutrients, and initiate a massive round of inflammation.[4]

- People often struggle to eat enough calories, leading to a metabolism slowdown over time, and the calories being consumed aren't nutrient dense.

- If you follow a non-keto diet, you'll have to eat fats and carbs together to make sure you get both of these important macronutrients. Mixing these two nutrients is a recipe for reacquiring all the fat you just burned during your fast.

Because of the drawbacks I list here, I recommend 2MAD, breaking your fast with a mini break-fast meal followed by a normal-size meal sixty to ninety minutes later.

lower-carb, higher monounsaturated fat–diet had much less belly fat than the group that ate the same number of calories but a lower percentage of monounsaturated fats. This group also showed an increase in adiponectin, just like with fasting. On the other hand, less olive oil led to quite an increase in fat around the middle and trunk.

Omega-3s, abundant in the Mediterranean diet, also have a powerful effect on, you guessed it, adiponectin. Giving adults just 2 grams of omega-3s over the course of three months raised adiponectin levels 44 percent.[5]

So, when we combine intermittent fasting and the Mediterranean diet, we get two parallel mechanisms activating adiponectin—and serious fat loss.

If You're Looking for ...	Consider ...	Keep in Mind ...
Maximum fat loss	Keto diet	✓ Extends the benefits of your fast ✓ Requires rigorous attention to carb intake ✓ Works well with plant-based diets
Muscle building	Non-keto diet	✓ Offers an opportunity to manipulate insulin spikes to your advantage ✓ Involves understanding the difference between high and low glycemic-load carbs and how each influences the body
A lighter environmental footprint	Plant-based diet	✓ May require more planning to ensure consuming a complete nutrient profile
A flexitarian option and belly fat loss	Mediterranean diet	✓ Rich in foods that actively support fasting

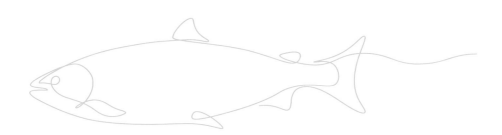

Sure, technically you can do intermittent fasting while eating any type of diet imaginable, but loading up on processed foods, sugar, and industrial vegetable oils (or the standard American diet) is going to make it harder for you to achieve your health and fitness goals and experience the full benefits of intermittent fasting. Eating whole, organic, non-GMO foods and reducing dairy, gluten, and sugar are just a few clean-eating basics that I recommend everyone follow to get the most nutrition in a limited timeframe.

Eating clean means having to work a little bit harder, but that modest investment will give you much more energy and power to achieve your health and fitness goals. Try it. I promise you will feel amazing.

Clean Eating Basics

EAT

✔ **WHOLE FOODS.** Fresh, from plants or animals, with minimal processing.

✔ **ORGANIC.** We want to limit exposure to synthetic herbicides, pesticides, and and other toxins that may have harmful effects on our body.[6] Choosing organic is a good way to avoid these unwanted substances while also supporting the environment. Organic foods are also:

(+) **Non-GMO foods.** Generally, plants and grains are genetically modified to make them more resistant to herbicides and pesticides and better able withstand harsher growing conditions. These chemicals are dangerous and we want to avoid, not ingest, them. Then, the modification process itself can create new proteins that our body doesn't recognize, causing our immune system to mount an attack against the unknown substances. This whole process does make it hard to find soy and corn, as these are two of the most common genetically modified crops. Buy organic fresh foods and look for packaged foods verified by the Non-GMO Project, an independent organization that only approves products with no genetically engineered ingredients whatsoever.

(+) **Hormone- and antibiotic-free foods (dairy, eggs, meat, etc.).** The antibiotics, hormones, and other chemicals fed to most commercially raised animals to promote faster growth and simply keep them alive may disrupt your endocrine system.[7] Labels can be deceptive, with requirements varying across foods and verification of claims weak. I recommend following the Environmental Working Group's (EWG) guidelines and look for foods certified by their "most reliable"

GRASS-FED, GRASS-FINISHED
MEAT TASTES BETTER

It's not just a marketing gimmick.
Grass-fed meat has a higher myofibrillar fat
content, meaning more little bits of fat throughout
the muscle fibers instead of big globs of fat, which
gives the meat more flavor.[8] And grass-fed meat has
higher amounts of naturally occurring glutamate, a
powerful neurotransmitter that is the source of our
fifth taste, umami. Go for grass-fed, grass-finished
for the health benefits and better taste.

organizations, such as the American Grassfed Association, Animal Welfare Approved, and the Marine Stewardship Council, who attest that no antibiotics were given to healthy animals and no synthetic growth hormones were used. Check out their label decoder (EWG.org/research/labeldecoder/) to dig deeper into this issue and shop responsibly.

✅ **GRASS-FED, GRASS-FINISHED MEATS.** Eating clean protein is imperative. You want to feed your body high-quality, naturally lean cuts of meat, not grain-fed garbage stuffed with extra fats, toxins, and pesticides. Grass-fed doesn't always mean grass-finished. Grass-fed just means that, at some point in that animal's lifetime, it ate grass.

✅ **SUSTAINABLY FISHED SEAFOOD,** low in mercury and toxins. Mercury from incinerators, mining operations, and power plants is a toxic metal that poisons our lakes, oceans, rivers, and streams. Large, older, or predatory fish have higher levels of mercury because it accumulates in their bodies over time. Symptoms of mercury exposure include dizziness, fatigue, irritability, memory and coordination problems, and numbness or tingling.[9] Chemicals, such as PCBs, dioxins, and DDT, leach into our waters from factories and industrial waste. Bottom-dwelling fish, including the American eel, sea trout, and wild striped bass, are the most susceptible to these toxins.[10] My top choices, for health benefits and my subjective sense of deliciousness, are:

→ **Wild Alaskan salmon:** high in vitamins B_3, B_6, B_{12}, and D and selenium and phosphorus

→ **Pacific sardines** (United States and Canada): high in omega-3 fatty acids, vitamins B_2, B_3, B_{12}, and D as well as calcium, copper, phosphorus, and selenium; plus it's inexpensive and easy to find canned

→ **Mussels:** high in vitamin B_{12} and iron, magnesium, omega-3s, phosphorus, potassium, and selenium

LIMIT

(-) PROCESSED FOODS. Some processed foods are better than others. There are many really good products on the market today made with minimally processed high-quality, clean ingredients. Their benefits, such as being easier to eat and store, outweigh the negatives for me. Others, not so much. The processed foods to keep away from are those that have little to no nutritional value or fiber and that are loaded with sugar, sodium, and chemicals you can barely pronounce (additives, artificial ingredients, fake flavorings, preservatives). Stay away from:

→ **Partially hydrogenated anything.** The hydrogenation process involves forcing hydrogen into a heated unsaturated liquid fat using a catalyst, such as nickel, to turn it into a shelf-stable soft-solid. The process also deodorizes and bleaches the fat to make it more palatable. Artificial trans fats, a health-hazardous form of unsaturated fat linked to an increased risk of insulin resistance and other associated conditions, are created during this process.[11]

→ **Anything reduced fat.** If the product is labeled "reduced fat," it means the manufacturer extracted the fat and then added something else to enhance the flavor.

(-) NATURAL SWEETENERS. You want to reduce *all* sugars. They're almost always empty calories that increase our cravings for more empty calories, edging out more nourishing, more satiating foods. When you need a little sweetness, opt for a little bit of stevia or monk fruit. Stevia is 300 times sweeter than table sugar and has been shown to lower blood glucose and improve glucose tolerance, whereas monk fruit, roughly 150 times sweeter than table sugar, does not affect insulin levels and may even have an antioxidant effect.[12]

(-) DAIRY. When casein, the dominant protein in cow's milk, is broken down, it releases beta-casomorphin 7 (BCM7), a peptide that is hard to break down and is inflammatory.[13] And, too much of the growth hormones naturally found in milk—no matter how organic and hormone-free it is—can throw off your hormones.[14] If you choose milk, go for raw goat's milk because the type of protein it contains does not break down into BCM7, so it is easier to digest, does not trigger an immune system response, and contains the healthy enzymes and probiotics pasteurized milk lacks.[15]

(-) ALCOHOL. Metabolizing alcohol asks a lot of your liver, the organ tasked with detoxifying and removing it from your blood. Alcohol breaks down into acetaldehyde, a substance so toxic it jumps the metabolism line, cutting ahead of every other type of food in your body so your liver can get it gone as quickly as possible. This sidelines other important bodily processes, including the metabolism of fats. Too much alcohol overwhelms the liver so it can't process the alcohol in a timely manner, causing a waterfall of damage to the liver (fatty liver, cirrhosis) and the rest of the body (central nervous system damage, dysregulated insulin, poor nutrient absorption). If your liver isn't healthy, you won't be able to burn fat efficiently, and if you're intermittent fasting to burn fat, well, you see the problem. If you're going to consume alcohol, keep it to a minimum, choose types that are easier on the system, such as vodka and gin, and only consume it after you've already absorbed some food.

AVOID

❌ **SUGAR AND ARTIFICIAL SWEETENERS.** Sugar is everywhere, especially in processed foods. It's addictive—and we eat way too much of it.[16] The average American consumes 13 to 16 percent of their total calories from added sugars, which equals about 32 teaspoons of added sugar daily! Consuming too much sugar is tied to many health problems, most notably insulin resistance, obesity, and chronic inflammation.[17] Sugar goes by many names—at least 61 different ones are listed on food labels, according to the University of California San Francisco—including many that end in "ose," such as sucrose, high fructose corn syrup, and dextrose, as well as barley malt and rice syrup.[18]

Artificial sweeteners, such as aspartame and saccharin, are synthetic sugar substitutes that may be calorie-free, or virtually so, but can still increase cravings, weight, and your risk of chronic conditions.[19] And although some natural sweeteners, such as raw honey and maple syrup, may contain antioxidants and prebiotics, sugar is sugar—and does your health or waistline no favors.

Need another reason to just say no? Sugar robs us of vitamins and minerals, inhibiting the absorption of magnesium, stealing vitamin C's ride into cells, and breaking down vitamin D. All of your good work undone.[20]

Avoid sugar. It's that simple.

❌ **HIGHLY PROCESSED SEED AND VEGETABLE OILS** high in omega-6 fatty acids. There is a concern that highly processed seed and vegetable oils are dangerous as they contain high amounts of omega-6s, and omega-6s are believed to promote inflammation. In rodent studies, omega-6s have been shown to be inflammatory, but this does not seem to be the case in humans. In short, the commonly consumed omega-6, linoleic acid, which accounts for 90% of omega-6 intake, has to be converted into arachidonic (ARA), and ARA promotes inflammation. However, it was found that in humans the enzyme delta-6 desatu-

TOP TACTIC

EAT THESE GRAINS

Buckwheat	Teff
Quinoa	Wild rice

rase is the rate-limiting enzyme that inhibits the conversion of LA to ARA.[21]

❌ **GLUTEN AND MOST GRAINS.** Gluten is not just an issue for people with celiac disease. Gluten causes a general immune response within the body because, over time, we've evolved into people who don't metabolize gluten well.[22] But, gluten isn't the only culprit. Other grains contain agglutinins, such as wheat germ agglutinin, which are proteins that cause red blood cells to glob together, and are very difficult to digest, stimulating the immune system and contributing to leaky gut. Agglutinins also block leptin, preventing this hormone released by fat cells from telling the brain that we have enough energy stored in our fat cells so we can rev up the metabolism.[23] Yes, you can store a lot more fat if you eat the wrong grains, which include barley, bulgur, corn, farro, spelt, oats, rice, rye, and wheat. (Even though oats don't contain gluten, the likelihood of cross-contamination at the farming and processing levels is very high.)

On Omegas: It's thought that a lot of the health concerns surrounding omega intake is more of a result of not consuming enough omega-3s. So while omega-6s may not be inflammatory in humans, omega-6 research is consistently evolving, and there may be more to the omega-3 vs. omega-6 dilemma. Omega-6s are not inherently "bad," but there is a large body of research suggesting omega-3s are a better option.[24] More information can be found on the National Center for Biotechnology Information or ScienceDirect websites.

Clean Eating Basics

Eat	Limit	Avoid
✓ Grass-fed, grass-finished, hormone- and antibiotic-free meats	✓ Alcohol	✓ Gluten and most grains
✓ Non-GMO foods	✓ Dairy	✓ Highly processed seed and vegetable oils
✓ Organic foods	✓ Natural sweeteners	✓ Sugar and artificial sweeteners
✓ Whole foods	✓ Processed foods	
✓ Sustainably fished seafood that is low in mercury and toxins		

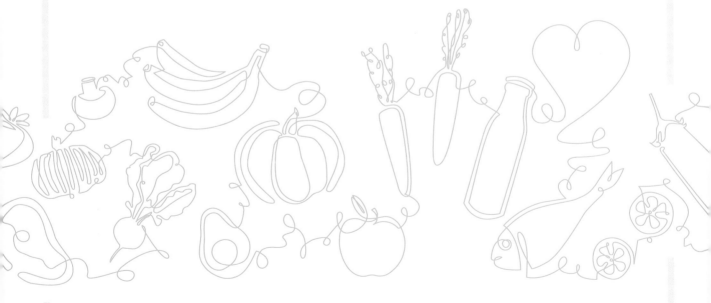

THE IMPORTANCE OF GETTING ENOUGH VITAMINS, MINERALS, AND GUT SUPPORT

If you're eating a well-rounded diet, you shouldn't have too many issues with vitamin and mineral deficiencies, but you may need to take extra care as you start intermittent fasting. Your eating window is smaller on certain days, meaning it's more challenging to get all the nutrients you need. Being aware of this and paying attention to where you may fall short can help.

I'm a big fan of trying to get nutrients from food (and, in the case of vitamin D, quality time spent outdoors) but, even with the best of plans, sometimes that's just too difficult, especially because intermittent fasting limits your available eating window. In this case, high-quality supplements are a good option to fill those gaps.

→ **Coenzyme Q10.** This is one of my favorite all-around supplements. Like a souped-up shuttle bus, coenzyme Q10 is ruthlessly efficient at transporting electrons from the food we eat to the electron receptors within our cells. A quicker, easier transfer is great for overall energy metabolism.[25] Coenzyme Q10 is also an antioxidant, neutralizing free radicals.

Supplements are readily available, but coenzyme Q10 is also found in a variety of foods, such as broccoli, cauliflower, and spinach, as well as fatty fish and organ meats (heart, kidney, liver).

Tips for Choosing a High-Quality Supplement

There are a lot of supplements out there and, due to limited industry oversight, many are made with low-quality, or even toxic, ingredients. Here's what to look for in a quality supplement:

- Reputable company: Look for peer-reviewed research to back up the manufacturer's claims, formulations, and dosages.

- Third-party testing: NSF/ANSI 173 certification assures that products are what they say they are on the label and don't contain potentially harmful levels of impurities, such as heavy metals or pesticides.

- Clean ingredients: Non-GMO with no added artificial flavorings, colorings, fillers, sugars, or other additives.

- Allergen-free: No dairy, gluten, or soy.

MEN: SUPPLEMENT WITH BORON

Boron is a trace mineral that unlocks, or frees, bound-up testosterone so you can use it. Most of the testosterone in our bodies, approximately 98 percent, is bound to sex hormone binding globulin (SHBG), a molecule tasked with transporting testosterone and other sex hormones throughout the body. A small amount of boron, about 6 to 9 mg each day, can increase free testosterone levels, promoting more muscle mass, overall energy, and strength.[26] You can also increase your dietary intake of boron by eating fruits and vegetables such as apples, avocados, cooked beans, peaches, pears, and even coffee.[27]

You do not want to take in too much boron, though, as it may become toxic at greater than 20 mg per day.

→ **Magnesium.** Very, very important for just about every enzymatic function in our body. Without enough magnesium, we can't create ATP, the energy currency that allows us to thrive, or balance our blood sugar.[28] That's right. One of magnesium's jobs is to modulate blood sugar. Magnesium and insulin have a reciprocal relationship. Insulin lets magnesium into the cell, and magnesium helps insulin do its job by processing glucose. Without enough magnesium, blood sugar levels go up and it takes more insulin to shuttle glucose into cells. Over time, low levels of magnesium can lead to insulin resistance.[29]

An electrolyte, *magnesium is okay to take during your fasting window*, but if you haven't gotten your recommended daily allowance yet, get it in now. Eat magnesium-rich foods such as avocados, Brazil nuts, chickpeas, flaxseed, lentils, salmon, and unsweetened dark chocolate.

→ **Omega-3 fatty acids.** Supporting protein absorption, lower inflammation, brain health, mood, and memory, omega-3s should be taken as part of breaking your fast, but you may also need supplementation later in your eating window to get a sufficient dose.[30] Vegans and vegetarians should pay particular attention as they tend to be low in omega-3s.[31] Except for sea veggies, plant foods do not contain sufficient quantities of eicosapentaenoic acid (EPA) and docosahexaenoic acid (DHA), two types of omega-3s. Fish and seafood are the best sources, so even omnivores who do not eat seafood are at risk of not getting enough DHA.

I like algal or calamarine oil (derived from squid or calamari) because the lower you go down the food chain, the more potent the omega-3s are.

→ **Probiotics.** As you may have already guessed, I am a big fan of gut bacteria. Probiotics add beneficial live bacteria to your gut. I recommend *Bacillus*-based probiotics because the *Bacillus* form spores that can actually make it to your colon, whereas many other probiotics are just killed by stomach acid. Fermented foods such as sauerkraut, pickles (not made with vinegar), kimchi, and high-quality yogurt are also good sources of probiotics.

→ **Vitamin B-complex.** You could take B-complex vitamins during your fasting window, but they can cause tummy trouble when taken on an empty stomach. I suggest supplementing during your eating window, instead. The vitamin B-complex is made up of eight B vitamins: B_1 (thiamine), B_2 (riboflavin), B_3 (niacin), B_5 (pantothenic acid), B_6 (pyridoxine), B_7 (biotin), B_9 (folic acid), and B_{12} (cobalamin). These vitamins are essential for a healthy body, as well as brain and nerve function, cell metabolism, good digestion, and energy levels. Eating a variety of fish, fruits, meats, and vegetables is the best way to bring more B vitamins into your diet.

Vegans and vegetarians are often B_{12} deficient because this vitamin is almost exclusively found in animal foods, including dairy, eggs, fish, and meats. Many plant milks and vegan processed foods are fortified with B_{12}; however, if you eat a whole foods diet that does not include consuming many processed foods (and I hope you are), you are at an especially high risk of deficiency. Nutritional yeast is one option, in addition to supplementation, to support B_{12} consumption. Two kinds of B_{12} supplements are vegan: cyanocobalamin and methylcobalamin. As mentioned previously, B_{12}, which helps maintain a healthy body, as well as brain and nerve function, cell metabolism, good digestion, and energy levels, is also involved in the making of DNA and red blood cells and linked to mood and memory.[32]

→ **Vitamin C.** Vitamin C does way more than help our immune cells function and stop us from getting sick. It's essential for the growth and repair of tissues throughout the body—from bones and cartilage to skin and blood vessels—and is a powerful antioxidant, preventing the damage caused by free radicals.

The body can't make vitamin C or store it. We have to get it from supplements or foods. Choose veggies such as bell peppers, broccoli, Brussels sprouts, kale, snow peas, and tomatoes. Why? Glucose competes with vitamin C for the same transport into the cell, and in that contest, vitamin C loses. If you take vitamin C with sugar or carbs (or think you're loading up by drinking orange juice), it won't get absorbed by the body.

→ **Vitamin D.** Getting enough vitamin D (for the record, a hormone) is important for everyone, and many of us are deficient. Even those of us who live in areas with a lot of sunlight where we can get outside and soak up the rays so our body can make vitamin D struggle to get enough. Your immune system requires vitamin D, and you need to have sufficient vitamin D to absorb calcium, which is critical for bone health. New research also suggests a link between low vitamin D and obesity, suggesting vitamin D's involvement in fat loss, especially belly fat.[33] If you're over age forty, vitamin D helps prevent sarcopenia, the muscle loss that naturally occurs with age.[34]

A bonus for everyone, though, is that vitamin D improves metabolism. One study published in the *European Journal of Nutrition* found that just a ten nanomole increase in vitamin D resulted in a thirteen calorie increase in metabolic rate.[35] That means for every ten nanomoles of vitamin D taken into the body, thirteen more calories are burned at rest. This result is likely due to the role vitamin D plays in improving musculoskeletal health, including muscle repair and recovery. Vitamin D will help keep your metabolism burning hot during your eating window.

Vegans and vegetarians are particularly vulnerable to vitamin D deficiency as the foods highest in vitamin D—egg yolks, salmon, and shellfish—aren't vegan friendly. Many plant milks and vegan processed foods are fortified with vitamin D, but I don't recommend a steady diet of these foods. Be sure to choose a vegan supplement, such as vitamin D_3, which is derived from lichen.

TOP TACTIC

WOMEN: MODULATE DAIRY

There is some evidence that the hormone rBST, which is found in cheeses, yogurt, and butter made from cows treated with it, triggers the production of IGF-1, a very important growth hormone for the development of the female mammary system.[36] (Milks are required to note on the label if they contain rBST, while other forms of dairy are not.) The gist? Excess dairy consumption may lead to higher amounts of IGF-1, which some research suggests could cause health concerns.[37] Be careful with dairy in general and make sure you are getting it from an organic source that you know does not contain rBST.

Micronutrient	Supports	Present In
Coenzyme Q10	✓ Antioxidant ✓ Overall energy metabolism	✓ Broccoli ✓ Cauliflower ✓ Fatty fish ✓ Organ meats ✓ Spinach
Magnesium	✓ Hundreds of biochemical reactions, including energy creation, muscle movements, and blood sugar regulation	✓ Avocados ✓ Brazil nuts ✓ Chickpeas ✓ Flaxseed ✓ Lentils ✓ Salmon ✓ Unsweetened dark chocolate
Omega-3 fatty acids	✓ Brain health ✓ Lower inflammation ✓ Memory ✓ Mood ✓ Protein absorption	✓ Seafood ✓ Sea veggies
Probiotics	✓ Gut microbiome	✓ Fermented foods ✓ Yogurt
B-complex vitamins	✓ Brain and nerve function ✓ Cell metabolism ✓ Energy levels ✓ Good digestion	✓ A variety of fish, fruits, meats, and vegetables
Vitamin C	✓ Antioxidant ✓ Growth and repair ✓ Immune system	✓ Bell peppers ✓ Broccoli ✓ Brussels sprouts ✓ Kale ✓ Snow peas ✓ Tomatoes
Vitamin D	✓ Bones and muscles ✓ Immune system	✓ Egg yolks ✓ Salmon ✓ Shellfish

How you approach your eating window definitely influences the results of your fast. These common mistakes can cost you dearly.

→ **Undereating.** Do not be afraid to eat during your eating window or on nonfasting days. Remember, the focus of intermittent fasting is not to shrink your caloric intake to achieve weight loss or any other benefit. Sure, day to day, your caloric intake might be lower on fasting days than it is on nonfasting days because you have a smaller window to consume calories, but big picture, say over the course of a week, it doesn't have to be all that different. The primary goal of intermittent fasting is to flip that metabolic switch so you start burning stored body fat and trigger a laundry list of physiological changes, such as autophagy, to optimize your body in a whole new way. So, don't think of your eating window as a period of time in which to eat like a bird. Eat your goal baseline level of calories during your eating window to try to offset the fact that you didn't consume calories during your fasting window. (If you're trying to lose weight, I recommend not reducing your baseline calories by more than 10 percent.) The changes in your body caused by fasting will help you lose fat; curbing calories won't.

If you slowly reduce your calories every day, your body will slow your metabolism to accommodate the lower amount of food coming in. It's called adaptive thermogenesis (*thermogenesis* meaning the creation of heat) because the amount of body heat created drops due to less food being available to create it. The contestants in *The Biggest Loser*, a weight-loss reality show and competition focused on eating less and exercising more, are perfect examples of how this happens. A study found that even six years after the show, contestants still had a metabolic rate of 700 calories fewer than it was before.[38] Losing weight via continual caloric restriction, whether through intermittent fasting or not, ultimately results in a slower metabolism and difficulty maintaining a healthy weight. Please, eat enough, and do not skimp on food during your eating window.

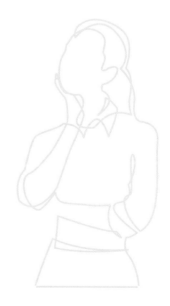

→ **Pushing meals too close to bedtime.** Our schedules are so packed that it may seem that the only time we have to eat is late at night after things have quieted down. Unfortunately, this is not a good plan. Your pancreas, the organ that secretes insulin in response to food, has melatonin receptors.[39] Melatonin is the hormone released when the sun goes down to signal it's time for sleep and restorative mode. When melatonin rises, the pancreas recognizes that signal and becomes a little less efficient at making insulin, regulating blood sugar levels, and utilizing and storing the foods you've consumed. You won't be getting the maximum benefit from your meal, and you'll be contributing to insulin resistance, making your fasts less effective.

I know it can be difficult, but try to break your fast close to 3:00 p.m. to 4:00 p.m. so you have enough time for your mini break-fast meal, normal-size meal, and any final snack by 7 p.m. Avoid eating too late in the day, or at night, when your melatonin levels are up.

CHECKLIST

EATING TO SUPPORT YOUR HEALTH AND FITNESS GOALS MADE EASY

Use this checklist to help ensure you're eating to support your health and wellness goals, and not inadvertently working against them.

☐ Consume a well-rounded, nutrient-dense diet filled with a variety of foods.

☐ Choose an eating style that matches your lifestyle, personal preferences, and health goals (not someone else's).

☐ Eat clean.

☐ Fill nutrient gaps with high-quality supplements.

☐ Support your microbiome with probiotics.

☐ Eat an adequate number of calories over the course of the week.

☐ Have your last meal before 7 p.m.

A solid eating style supports your body full time and makes intermittent fasting easier and more powerful. Knowing how to address possible mineral deficiencies and snacking will set you on the right path.

How do I know if I have a vitamin or mineral deficiency?

Some of the most common symptoms indicating your body is not getting all the nutrients it needs include:

→ Brittle hair and nails

→ Fatigue

→ Hair loss

→ Mouth ulcers or cracks in the corners of the mouth

→ Muscle cramps

→ Numbness or tingling

→ Skin problems

But, how do you determine exactly which nutrient you're lacking? It can be tricky to pinpoint a specific vitamin or mineral deficiency on your own, as each has its own set of symptoms, and many overlap. Contact your health care provider, who can review your diet and order blood tests to figure out where you need more support. These blood work results can also act as a helpful baseline to monitor going forward.

Is it okay to snack throughout my eating window or on nonfasting days?

Just say no to grazing. Quit the six-meals-a-day thing and eating mindlessly or out of habit. Stick with three meals per day on nonfasting days. Look: Those "little" bits and bites of food here and there add up to a lot of extra calories and pounds of fat. Avoiding snacks will also help keep your insulin levels stable throughout the day. Every time we eat, we spike our insulin, and when our insulin spikes, our body goes into storage mode. The more frequently we eat, the fewer opportunities we have to burn fat.

A study published in the journal *Diabetologia* found that subjects with type 2 diabetes who ate two larger meals each day ended up burning more fat than subjects who ate six smaller meals, even though both groups ate the same number of calories and macronutrients.[40] Not apples to apples in this case because I'm not telling you to eat only two meals a day, but keep in mind, if you're grazing throughout the day, grabbing a few nuts between meals, you're turning off your fat-burning system.

LET'S BREAK IT DOWN

- Intermittent fasting works with any eating style, but some, such as keto, non-keto, plant-based, and Mediterranean, offer unique benefits that can help you reach your goals more quickly.

- No matter which style of eating you choose, make sure you get adequate nutrients through foods and fill gaps with high-quality supplements.

- Focus on fresh, whole, organic foods that are non-GMO and hormone- and antibiotic-free. Look for grass-fed, grass-finished meats and seafood that is sustainably fished and low in mercury and toxins.

- Avoid sugar, highly processed seed and vegetable oils, gluten, and most grains.

- Don't undereat or snack during your eating window or on nonfasting days. Focus on triggering the metabolic switch that will start burning stored fat instead of significantly shrinking your calorie intake, and stick with two or three meals each day rather than grazing.

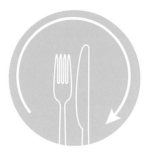

CHAPTER 7

Tool Kit

The tools covered in this chapter will help make intermittent fasting even easier. Use them alongside the guidelines and checklists in the previous chapters.

SAMPLE FASTING SCHEDULES

You'll find schedules for:

→ Twelve-hour fast (12:12)

→ Sixteen-hour fast (16:8), skipping breakfast

→ Sixteen-hour fast (16:8), skipping dinner

→ Twenty-hour fast (20:4), skipping dinner

These sample schedules will give you an idea of how the timing of a fast can look. As you'll see, it's easy to adjust the starting time of your fasting window but keep these key elements in mind as you do:

→ When you prefer to workout

→ When you'll break your fast and eat your normal-size meal, preferably before 7 p.m.

Sample Twelve-Hour Fasting Schedule (12:12)

The twelve-hour fast is a good way to dip your toe into fasting. A popular schedule is to fast from 7 p.m. to 7 a.m. so most of your fasting window is open while you sleep. Nice! Just wake-up, workout, and break your fast right after.

If you want to start getting into the rhythm of what fasting feels like during the day and you are an early riser, try the following.

FASTING WINDOW: 6 A.M. TO 6 P.M.

6 a.m.	Begin fast
6:30 a.m.	Apple cider vinegar drink
At least 7 a.m.	Caffeinated fasting-friendly beverage (optional)
1 p.m.	Switch to noncaffeinated fasting-friendly beverages
4:30 to 5:30 p.m.	Work out
5:30 p.m.	Cinnamon + salt + magnesium to lower cortisol
6 p.m.	Mini break-fast meal: fasting window now closed
7 p.m. to 7:30 p.m.	Normal-size meal

Sample Sixteen-Hour Fasting Schedule (16:8), Skipping Breakfast

FASTING WINDOW: 7 P.M. TO 11 A.M.

7 p.m.	Begin fast
9 p.m.	Apple cider vinegar drink ➜ Go to bed
7 a.m.	Wake up
7:30 a.m	Apple cider vinegar drink
7:30 a.m. to 8:30 a.m.	Work out
8:30 a.m.	Caffeinated fasting-friendly beverage (optional), then switch to noncaffeinated fasting-friendly beverages for the remainder of the fasting window
10:30 a.m.	Cinnamon + salt + magnesium to lower cortisol
11 a.m.	Mini break-fast meal: fasting window now closed
12 p.m. to 12:30 p.m.	Normal-size meal

Sample Sixteen-Hour Fasting Schedule (16:8), Skipping Dinner

FASTING WINDOW: 5 P.M. TO 9 A.M.

5 p.m.	Begin fast
9 p.m.	Apple cider vinegar drink → Go to bed
7 a.m.	Wake up
7:30 a.m.	Apple cider vinegar drink
7:30 a.m. to 8:30 a.m	Work out
8:30 a.m.	Cinnamon + salt + magnesium to lower cortisol
9 a.m.	Mini break-fast meal: fasting window now closed
10 a.m. to 10:30 a.m.	Normal-size meal

Sample Twenty-Hour Fasting Schedule (20:4), Skipping Dinner

FASTING WINDOW: 1 P.M. TO 9 A.M.

1 p.m.	Begin fast
9 p.m.	Apple cider vinegar drink → Go to bed
7 a.m.	Wake up
7:30 a.m.	Apple cider vinegar drink
7:30 a.m. to 8:30 a.m.	Work out
8:30 a.m.	Cinnamon + salt + magnesium to lower cortisol
9 a.m.	Mini break-fast meal: fasting window now closed
10 a.m. to 10:30 a.m.	Normal-size meal

SELF-ASSESSMENT: ARE YOU GETTING THE MOST FROM INTERMITTENT FASTING?

Use this quiz as a way to check your progress. If you've been intermittent fasting for at least one month but are not seeing the results you expected, or if you just think something's "off," this assessment will identify where you may be going wrong and get you back on track or direct you to the next chapters to amplify if that's what you need next.

Answer the following questions:

1. Are you experiencing the results you are looking for from intermittent fasting?
___ Yes   ___ No

2. Are you losing weight?
___ Yes   ___ No

3. Are you comfortable fasting for your desired fasting length?
___ Yes   ___ No

4. Are you able to manage hunger easily during your fasting window?
___ Yes   ___ No

5. Do you feel mentally sharp during your fasting window?
___ Yes   ___ No

6. Do you feel energized immediately following a fast?
___ Yes   ___ No

7. Is your digestion good, with daily bowel movements and no bloating, constipation, diarrhea, or gas?
___ Yes   ___ No

8. Are you clear of dry mouth, fatigue, headaches, and muscle cramps?
___ Yes   ___ No

9. Have you found ways to incorporate stress-relieving relaxation techniques into your daily life?
___ Yes   ___ No

If you answered "Yes" to:

0 TO 3 QUESTIONS: Don't be discouraged! Getting the hang of intermittent fasting can take time and practice. Be patient with yourself. Read about what may not be going as planned in the explanations following and return to chapters 4, 5, and 6 for a refresher on the basics. Give yourself at least another month with those refinements in place and retake the quiz.

4 TO 6 QUESTIONS: Congratulations! You're on the right track and experiencing some of the benefits of intermittent fasting. With a few tweaks, your results could be even better. Read the explanations following for those questions you answered "No" to and learn how to turn those Nos into Yeses. Try a few more weeks of intermittent fasting with that troubleshooting locked in and then retake the quiz.

7 TO 9 QUESTIONS: You've got this! You're ready to take intermittent fasting to the next level and try additional strategies to amplify your fast. Fix any lingering trouble spots with the following guidance and then get going on part 3.

If you answered "No" to:

QUESTION #1: You may be consuming something inadvertently during your fasting window that is breaking your fast so you don't actually ever get into a fasting state. The best way to avoid this is to keep it super simple and go back to basics: only water, black coffee, and plain tea during your fasting window. Also:

➜ Make sure you break your fast properly and, again, go back to basics and try breaking your fast with lean protein only.

➜ If you fast more than three times each week, try cutting back to one or two days. Fasting too frequently and slowing your metabolism is a common reason for no, or stalled, results.

➜ Are you comfortable at your current fasting length and confident you're ticking all the boxes on the checklists in the previous three chapters? Try extending your fast. You may need more time to get into a fat-burning state.

QUESTION #2: A lack of weight loss is usually the result of:

➜ Fasting too frequently. By fasting more than three times each week, you're likely not eating enough each day, inadvertently reducing your caloric intake and slowing your metabolism. Limit your fasting to two days each week and make sure you're eating enough, especially on nonfasting days, to see if your results change.

➜ Eating too much during your eating window. Being hungry while fasting can make it hard to break your fast in moderation and lead to bingeing. Incorporate satiating foods and drinks into your pre-fast, fasting, and post-fasting routine (chapter 4 has suggestions).

➜ Difficulty fasting for at least sixteen hours. If pushing your fasting time to sixteen hours or beyond is a pain point, go back to a fasting length that felt good to you, even if that's ten hours, and slowly add one hour every week, so your body acclimates to fasting, and slowly extend your fasting window. You want to feel confident and comfortable at each fasting length before adding more time. Use satiating foods and drinks during your pre-fast, fasting, and post-fasting routine (chapter 4 has suggestions) for extra support.

QUESTION #3: You may have pushed your fasting length too far, too fast. Try a shorter fasting length for a few weeks, slowly adding more time to your fasting window. Your body could need extra time to acclimate to fasting. In addition:

→ If hunger is an obstacle, add satiating foods and drinks during your pre-fast, fasting, and post-fasting routine (chapter 4 has suggestions) to help make fasting for longer lengths of time more manageable.

→ Hydrate, hydrate, hydrate.

→ Manage your stress, especially on fasting days, by using deep breathing, taking a walk outside, or doing a few quick stretches.

QUESTION #4: Adding satiating foods and drinks into your pre-fast, fasting, and post-fasting routine (chapter 4 has suggestions) will help. Remember, feelings of hunger can be a conditioned response from years and years of habit. Eating breakfast every morning at 8 a.m. sets you up to feel hungry every morning at 8 a.m., even if your body isn't actually in need of refueling yet. Simply seeing and smelling food—and food is everywhere!—can make you hungry, no matter how nourished your body may be. It can take a while to break these habits and conditioned responses.

During your fasting window, add new habits to replace old ones. Always eat breakfast at 8 a.m.? Have a fasting-friendly beverage at that time instead. Easing the grip of these hunger-generating conditioned responses will not only make fasting easier, but it will also make it easier for you to hear when your body is truly hungry. Another tip: Be busy. Keep your mind and body active and you'll be focused on the task at hand, not hunger.

QUESTION #5: Dehydration and a lack of electrolytes are common culprits. Be sure to drink plenty of water and add those electrolytes—sodium, magnesium, and potassium—during your fasting window.

QUESTION #6: After a fast, your body is ramping up a lot of systems that have been in low gear—and that takes energy. Supporting your body with proteolytic digestive enzymes, coenzyme Q10, and bee propolis when you break your fast should give you an added boost.

QUESTION #7: Support your gut and ease symptoms of distress by limiting your fast to a maximum of three times each week. If you're really struggling, cut your schedule to two fasting days. In the short-term, fasting weakens the gut, and if you're fasting too much and not adequately supporting your gut health, it won't rebuild. This leads me to highlight some of the ways to make sure you promote a healthy gut mucosal layer and microbiome:

→ Drink green tea before and during your fast.

→ Break your fast properly to avoid irritating your gut.

→ Include prebiotics and probiotics in your diet.

Chapters 4, 5, and 6 include even more suggestions for maintaining gut health. Yep, your gut is that important.

QUESTION #8: These are common signs of dehydration. The color of your urine is another indication. You want a light straw color, nothing too dark or concentrated. I can't emphasize enough how important adequate hydration is: hydrate, hydrate, hydrate. Add fasting-friendly flavorings (a slice of lemon, a dash of ground cinnamon) to water, brew some green tea, and keep your water bottle or thermos near you throughout the day.

QUESTION #9: What are you waiting for? You don't need to dedicate a lot of time to lowering stress and promoting relaxation. Finding moments throughout your day to take a breather, laugh, romp with your kids or pets, journal, do a few sun salutations, give a loved one a hug, or walk around the block, will make fasting—and just about everything—that much easier and more manageable.

TOP TACTIC

TRUST YOUR GUT

Quizzes and self-assessments can only tell you so much, and they can't replace what you know deep down: whether or not you're physically and mentally ready to kick up your fasting a notch. I'm a big believer in a gut check, so do one now and listen to what it tells you.

Part 3

AMPLIFY YOUR RESULTS

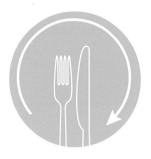

CHAPTER 8

Supercharge Fat Burning

So, you've got the basics down and are ready to accelerate your results. Try these strategies to increase fat burning. The point, though, isn't to try them all at once. Give one or two suggestions a go for a few weeks and see if they boost your results. If not, incorporate another one or two, and so on, until you find what works best for you—then do something else! Keeping it fresh is what makes intermittent fasting effective—and so not boring.

MIX THINGS UP

It's time to throw a wrench in things! You think you've got this intermittent fasting thing down pat? Well, it's time to switch it up! Try a new strategy to see new results. I am always experimenting on myself—mixing up my fasting lengths, schedule, workouts, you name it. I keep a calendar to help me track everything. You don't need to go as all-in on the experimenting as I do, but mixing up your routine is an easy way to amplify your results, especially when it comes to losing body fat. You want to keep your body guessing. Remember, many of the benefits of intermittent fasting come from shocking the body into the type of sporadic and spontaneous caloric reduction that causes the metabolic switch to flip from burning glucose to burning fat. Some ways to switch it up are:

→ Skip dinner instead of breakfast (or vice versa) and change up those options throughout the week/month.

→ Vary your fasting lengths throughout the week/month.

→ Work out at a different time, alternating between morning and evening workouts.

→ Try a new workout and be sure to vary your routines.

Additionally, I recommend spicing things up by:

→ **Adding a 5- to 10-minute HIIT (high-intensity interval training) workout.** A brief high-intensity workout triggers a significant rise in catecholamines (epinephrine and norepinephrine), hormones that drive fat burning. One study found the increase to be significant, with epinephrine increasing 6.3-fold and norepinephrine increasing 14.5-fold at the end of ten 6-second sprints interspersed with thirty seconds of recovery.[1] In contrast, steady-state aerobic exercise resulted in small increases of each. And guess what? With each sprint, more catecholamines were released. Epinephrine, in particular, drives the release of fat from muscle and subcutaneous fat (the fat beneath your skin), and there are more epinephrine receptors in the abdomen than anywhere else in the body. You have the potential to burn some serious belly fat by combining a quick HIIT session with intermittent fasting.

→ **Spending time in a sauna during your fasting window.** High heat is another way to stress the body, initiating the release of heat-shock proteins, protective molecules that help scavenge free radicals and chaperone amino acids.[2] By making sure amino acids get where they need to go, heat-shock proteins help preserve muscle, and more muscle means more metabolism, and more metabolism means more fat burning during your fast. The news is even better for women: One study found that thirty minutes in a sauna dramatically increased the amount of free fatty acids available in the bloodstream to be burned. This is likely due to higher levels of epinephrine, which doubled after sauna exposure, and a woman's increased sensitivity to epinephrine.[3] The perfect combination: Do your HIIT workout, then hit the sauna!

EXTEND YOUR FASTING WINDOW

If you feel great after fasting for twenty hours, you're ready to give prolonged fasting a shot. I've always been a big fan of sprinkling in a few longer-term fasts over the course of a month, or several months for a more aggressive result. A longer fast gives your body extra time to utilize fat as a fuel source.

After about sixteen hours, your body runs out of stored carbs and starts to generate more energy from gluconeogenesis, the creation of glucose from body fat and protein.[4] At sixteen hours, we have a big improvement in our potential fat loss. The demand for glucose, primarily from the brain, stays fairly aggressive up until about twenty-eight hours. This means the demand to turn body fat into glucose is very high. Between sixteen and twenty-eight hours is the fat burning sweet spot—a peak fat burning period. If you extend your fast longer, your body will shift again, from making glucose for energy through gluconeogenesis to making ketones for energy through ketogenesis. Ketones are made from the breakdown of fat, so the utilization of fat as an energy source continues.

By getting your body used to extended fasts, you add another fat-loss tool to your intermittent fasting toolbox. The longer the fast, the more infrequently you should do them, and breaking a prolonged fast and other considerations are different. (For resources on how to fast longer, visit FastingIsEasy.com.) Here are some fasting length options:

WHOLE-DAY FASTING (TWENTY-FOUR HOURS). A personal favorite, with studies showing amazing fat loss and overall weight loss of between 3 and 9 percent with twenty-four-hour fasting one or two days each week.[5] If you're interested in losing a lot of weight, not just toning up, whole-day fasting is worth trying. Especially if you don't want to spend a lot of time and effort thinking about fasting and eating windows during your day. Just focus on fasting for one twenty-four-hour period, once or twice each week, and you're good to go.

THIRTY-SIX-HOUR FAST. By thirty-six hours, you should be in ketosis and torching fat. A study published in *Cell Metabolism* looked at thirty-six-hour fasts. They had participants do these fasts more than one time per week, not at all what I would recommend, but the study is still a compelling look at the body composition benefits of this type of fast. Participants were divided into two groups. One group fasted for

If you want to burn fat and you're not working out in a fasted state, you really, really should be. A study published in the *British Journal of Nutrition* tracked two groups of individuals. One group fasted before a 10 a.m. workout whereas the other group had breakfast before working out. Both groups did the same workout and drank the same chocolate protein shake post-workout. A few hours later, both groups were offered a pasta lunch and instructed to eat until they felt "comfortably full." The fasted group burned 20 percent more fat than the nonfasted group. And, for those who think exercising on an empty stomach would make you eat more later to make up for it, think again. The fasted group did not eat any more pasta than the other group.[6]

Alternate-Day Fasting

This type of fasting is just what it sounds like: alternating twenty-four hours of fasting with twenty-four hours of nonfasting. So, one day on, one day off.

It's an intense approach to fasting but also a very effective way to lose fat. In one meta-analysis comparing the results of twenty-one different fasting studies with fasting lengths of between sixteen and twenty hours, whole day, and alternate day, alternate-day fasting resulted in the best fat loss, at 6.6 to 12 pounds (3 to 5.5 kg) in trials from three to twelve weeks.[7] That's some aggressive burn.

My concern with alternate-day fasting as a standard practice is the potential long-term impact on your metabolism. It's tough to get all of your caloric needs met with such a limited eating window and, if you're regularly eating fewer calories, your metabolism will slow to compensate.

Alternate-day fasting takes a lot of discipline to do—and to do it right–but if you're a hyperdisciplined person, motivated to get the maximum amount of fat loss possible, it's very effective. Sustainable? Not so much. I suggest using it to lose the last 10 to 15 pounds (4.5 to 6.8 kg), then switching to a more sustainable fasting schedule.

thirty-six hours, ate whatever they wanted in unlimited amounts for twelve hours, and then started another thirty-six-hour fast. The second group could eat whatever they wanted, as much as they wanted, but were told not to try to gain or lose weight. Researchers found that the fasting group lost 7.7 pounds (3.5 kg) and didn't really overeat that much on their eating days.[8] Pretty impressive. Even more impressive? On eating days, the fasting group participants had elevated levels of ketones, meaning this thirty-six-hour fast has a benefit that extends over multiple days. A thirty-six-hour fast is my personal sweet spot. I do one at least every three or four months.

FORTY-EIGHT-HOUR FAST. The big benefits come from the fact that you get deeply into ketosis and burning fat to create massive amounts of ketones. Fat loss during a forty-eight-hour fast is supreme. I do forty-eight-hour fasts at least once every couple months. It's the perfect reset. After forty-eight hours, I start to worry about some muscle atrophy and the impact that can have on your metabolism, so max out here if your focus is creating a large fat-burning effect.

EXTEND YOUR FAST WITHOUT FASTING

Use fasting-mimicking foods to get the benefits of a long fast without actually having to fast. Let's say you want to do a twenty-four-hour fast but have trouble after the twenty-hour mark. By consuming fasting mimicking-foods (and other fasting-friendly foods) for four hours, you could turn that twenty-hour fast into a whole-day fast. Perfect? No. The only true way to get the most out of a twenty-four-hour fast (or any fasting length) is to do the fast, but you will see gains. Fair warning: You won't be making beautiful, gourmet meals with these ingredients. If you manage that, reach out with your recipes!

These foods continue to turn down growth signaling:

- ✓ Algal and cod liver oil
- ✓ Flax
- ✓ Macadamia nuts
- ✓ MCT oil
- ✓ Olives
- ✓ Pure unsweetened dark chocolate

While these foods induce autophagy:

- ✓ Ginger
- ✓ Green tea
- ✓ Rishi
- ✓ Turmeric

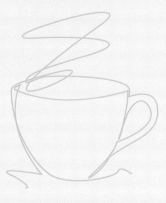

Accelerate fat burning by getting into a fasted state quickly. You'll get more out of your fast without having to spend more time fasting. We've covered some foods that can help with this already, including:

→ Apple cider vinegar
→ Caffeine
→ Cayenne pepper
→ Ginger
→ Lemon verbena tea
→ Mediterranean spices
→ Turmeric

The right combination of foods can do a lot to promote fat burning, as can the right movement. Consider the keto diet and a workout to support your lymph system.

Keto Diet

Intermittent fasting and the keto diet work together harmoniously because they both encourage the body to get into a highly efficient fat-burning state. Due to the metabolic shift that your body undergoes when you keep carbs low and fats high, your body begins pulling from its own fat stores to produce the energy it needs, resulting in weight loss. A study published in the journal *Diabetic Medicine* looked at the effectiveness of weight loss in a low-fat group versus a low-carb group. Because there are a lot of studies showing the effectiveness in normal individuals, this study actually looked at the effectiveness in type 2 diabetics and found that over a three-month period the keto group lost 15.2 pounds (6.9 kg), whereas the low-fat group lost only 4.6 pounds (2 kg). The keto diet caused three times more weight loss.[9]

On the keto diet, your body gets used to using fats as fuel, so when you do go into your fasting period, your body has the ability to switch gears and start burning fat quickly and efficiently and get you into ketosis much faster. By combining keto with intermittent fasting, you're kicking yourself into the optimal fasting state much more quickly and will start reaping the body composition, longevity, and other benefits much sooner.

To get started, I follow a strict keto diet for three to four weeks while putting a pause on fasting. For those weeks, focus on following a traditional keto diet and creating ketones to get your body fat adapted. After about a month, begin intermittent fasting again, two to three times each week.

Add an Upper/Lower Split Workout with a Twist

Usually, a workout routine divides training days between upper- and lower-body sessions. The upper/lower split workout I suggest starts with the lower body and then moves to the upper body, and both workouts are done during the same session, on the same day. It's an unconventional way to work out, but the reason it works has to do with the lymphatic system, a network of lymph vessels and lymph nodes that carry a fluid, lymph, from tissues around the body and into the blood.[10] It's completely separate from the circulatory system of blood vessels carrying blood to and from the heart.

Lymph is made mostly of white blood cells with a little bit of water, salts, protein, and glucose. Its jobs are to carry lymph around our immune system, bathe the cells of all of our tissues in nutrients, and shuttle bad things, such as bacteria and viruses, away. Lymph also transports fat before it reaches your bloodstream. To supercharge fat burning, we want to mobilize fat as much as possible during our fasting window. Here's where my unconventional workout comes in.

Our lymph system starts in the legs and works its way up. It also relies on muscle contraction to move lymph through the system. Every time you flex a muscle, you manually move lymph around. By pumping the muscles in your lower body and then your upper body, you transport lymph all the way up to the thoracic ducts, large veins on the left and right side of your neck, and into the bloodstream so fat can be delivered to the liver and be metabolized that much faster.[11] With this workout, you manually assist the mobilization of fat and get deeper into your fast.

TOP TACTIC

FOAM ROLLING AND AEROBIC EXERCISE

1. **Use a foam roller** to mobilize lymph and fat to accelerate fat burning while increasing blood flow, reducing inflammation, and promoting relaxation. Start with your lower body (calves, hamstrings, quads) and progress to your upper body (IT band, upper back, lats).

2. **Run, jump rope, stair climb, or bike.** Steady-state aerobic exercise increases lymph flow two to three times more than when at rest.[12]

TRY THESE SUPPLEMENTS

The following supplements will improve the effectiveness of your fast and help you burn more fat by supporting your body's stress response (remember, we want a fast to be stressful to the body so it adapts and grows stronger) or allowing you to perform a little bit better so you use up more fat for energy.

Tyrosine
Okay to take during your fasting window. Tyrosine, an amino acid, is a precursor to epinephrine and norepinephrine, the catecholamines that spike during a fast and initiate fat burning and loss. When these catecholamines are elevated, we experience all the benefits of

In addition to preventing catecholamine depletion, tyrosine supports cognitive flexibility, the ability to switch between thoughts or tasks, and overall cognitive function.[13] A precursor to dopamine, tyrosine is also linked to a balanced mood and sense of well-being, helping us manage stress better and stay focused.

a fast—but here's the thing: We can run out of them. If we do, we don't get as much out of the fast or use as much body fat for fuel as when they are present and elevated. Supplementing with tyrosine ensures the body has the raw material required to produce the epinephrine and norepinephrine we need.[14] When choosing a supplement, go for straight-up tyrosine (L-tyrosine), a more bioavailable option than N-acetyl L-tyrosine (NAT).

Creatine

Okay to take during your fasting window. Creatine, essentially, is an energy booster that supports the creation of ATP, the body's main energy currency. When we have reserves of creatine in our body, we can make ATP twelve times faster than without it and be better able to meet our body's energy needs without fatigue.[15]

The goal of supplementing with creatine is to build up and maintain your stores over time rather than as a one-off supplement here and there.

Essential Amino Acids (EAAs)

Do NOT take essential amino acids during your fasting window as they will break your fast. Instead, take them with your mini breakfast meal of high-quality protein. Essential amino acids are those that the body cannot make and that must be obtained through diet. There are nine essential amino acids: histidine, isoleucine, leucine, lysine, methionine, phenylalanine, threonine, tryptophan, and valine. These amino acids, and most especially leucine, are potent activators of mTOR, the driver of protein synthesis and muscle building.[16] More muscle equals more fat burning.

The Difference Between EAA and BCAA Supplements

Your body needs twenty different amino acids, and of these, nine are not able to be manufactured by the body and, so, must be consumed. These nine are called "essential amino acids" (EAAs). Branched-chain amino acids (BCAAs) are a group of three essential amino acids: isoleucine, leucine, and valine.

The takeaway: BCAA supplements contain only three EAAs, whereas EAAs contain all nine the body needs.

LET'S BREAK IT DOWN

- Keep your fasting routine fresh by mixing up fasting lengths, schedules, and workouts regularly.

- Try extending the length of your fast to twenty-four hours and beyond.

- Use fasting-mimicking foods, the keto diet, and/or lymph-stimulating workouts to mobilize fat.

- Add supplements, such as tyrosine, creatine, and EEAs, to help you burn more body fat for energy.

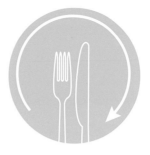

CHAPTER 9

Crush Inflammation

Chronic inflammation is bad for us. It's at the root of weight gain (and an inability to lose weight) and the root of why we flat out don't feel like ourselves anymore.[1] Inflammation taxes your immune system, halts fat loss and muscle building, and zaps cognitive function. It leaves you *drained*. And, when you're fatigued or not feeling your best, you won't be motivated to eat a healthy diet or work out. Reducing the amount of unnecessary inflammation in your body will give you the energy you need to live a healthy lifestyle and make good choices. Intermittent fasting will reduce inflammation, but here's what else you can do to power down inflammation even more and power up your fasting results.[2]

EXTEND YOUR FAST

Lengthening your fast to twenty-four, thirty-six, or even forty-eight hours gives you the anti-inflammatory benefits of a massive amount of ketones for a longer period of time. Ketones, first produced during gluconeogenesis, then later in your fast when your body switches mainly to ketogenesis, have been shown to dramatically decrease inflammatory markers within the body.

Several studies link ketones to blocking the NLRP3 inflammasome, a set of proteins released in response to infections or cell damage. The NLRP3 inflammasome works to nullify the threat and put your body in a stand-by mode that leaves you feeling tired and rundown. In one study, the ketone beta-hydroxybutyrate (BHB) was found to decrease those markers.[3] Now, of course, we want NLRP3 inflammasome working when we're sick—but when we're not sick, we definitely don't want it. With longer-term fasting, we fight low-grade chronic inflammation sapping our energy and resetting our immune system.[4]

Try a longer-term fast every few months and hit a big reset button on inflammation. (Visit FastingIsEasy.com for resources on how to fast longer.)

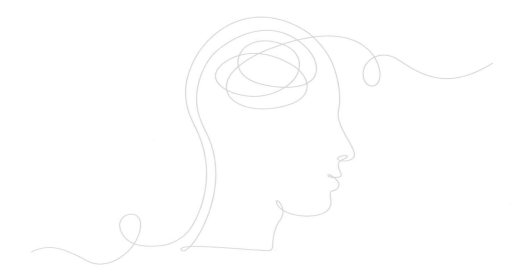

Poor gut health is a major contributor to chronic inflammation. A weak gut lining allows bacteria, food particles, and other stuff that should stay sealed up in the intestines to leak into the bloodstream. The immune system—a massive proportion of which is actually located in your digestive tract—recognizes these particles as pathogens and goes to work fighting them. A continuously compromised gut barrier kindles low-grade inflammation. The best thing we can do to prevent leaky gut and a full-scale immune system response is to support our gut mucosal layer.

Eliminate Inflammatory Foods

Inflammatory foods are linked to increased gut permeability and changes to the microbiome that can break down intestinal barriers. Avoiding inflammatory foods increases the stability and structure of your gut mucosal layer. Some of the most inflammatory foods are ones that will sound familiar, as I've already recommended avoiding them: A1 dairy, alcohol, gluten, high fructose corn syrup (read: processed foods), sugar, trans fats, and vegetable and seed oils.

Hand in hand with avoiding these inflammatory foods is identifying the foods that cause an inflammatory response in *your* body. Each body is unique and, to significantly knock back inflammation long term, cut out the foods that provoke an immune system response or digestive distress in you. Whether the food causes an allergic response driven by the immune system (hives, itching, swelling) or digestive-related symptoms (bloating, cramping, diarrhea, gas, nausea) suggesting a food sensitivity or intolerance, damage is being done. Some of the most likely culprits include:

→ Citrus
→ Eggs
→ Fish
→ Nightshades (tomatoes, potatoes, peppers, eggplant)
→ Peanuts
→ Sesame
→ Shellfish
→ Soybeans
→ Tree nuts

You're likely aware if you have a food allergy. The physical response is immediate and, usually, severe. Food sensitivities, on the other hand, can be harder to pinpoint, often because we tend to accept stomach discomfort as "normal" or "just the way it is." Don't.

Doing an elimination diet, a process that removes certain foods from your diet, for a set period of time before adding them back, one at a time, while monitoring your reaction, is the best way to tune in to your sensitivities and experience how good you can feel when inflammatory foods are out of the picture. An elimination diet takes effort, but it's worth it, to give your digestive system a break and get to the root of a significant source of inflammation.

Eat Anti-Inflammatory Foods

You could find pretty much any food out there and argue that some component of it is anti-inflammatory, even when it really isn't. A candy bar, for example, has chocolate in it, but that doesn't make it anti-inflammatory, does it? The following are truly potent anti-inflammatories in seven food categories: protein, vegetable, fruit, dairy, beverage, fat, and spice.

PROTEIN: SALMON

Salmon is high in omega-3s that are really powerful when it comes to inflammation modulation, inhibiting nuclear factor-kB (NF-kB), one of the main control towers for inflammation in our bodies, and converting it into anti-inflammatory resolvins.[5] Salmon actually changes the way the body responds to inflammation, cutting off the signal at the source. But salmon is special because it also contains astaxanthin, a powerful antioxidant that gives salmon its pinkish color. It has a free radical oxygen capacity 6,000 times that of vitamin C, meaning it can neutralize many more free radicals, and it's an epic multitasker, able to neutralize twenty free radical compounds at a time.[6] Most antioxidants have the ability to neutralize one to three. The combination of omega-3s and astaxanthin in salmon make it a top anti-inflammatory choice.

VEGETABLE: BEETS

Beets contain betanin and vulgaxanthin, two phytonutrients that reduce inflammation by inhibiting COX enzymes that are known

TOP TACTIC

DRINK BEET JUICE BEFORE A WORKOUT

Looking for better performance? A double-blind study published in the *Journal of Applied Physiology* found that people who consumed beet juice before a workout lasted 16 percent longer in their workouts compared to when given a placebo of blackcurrant cordial—so it's a pretty impressive result.[7] Researchers aren't entirely sure of the mechanism but suspect the nitrate contained in beet juice leads to a reduction in oxygen uptake, making exercise less tiring and boosting stamina at the same time.

to trigger inflammation.[8] Aspirin is an anti-inflammatory because it inhibits this same COX enzyme. Beets are also a good source of betaine, a nutrient that helps protect cells from environmental stress with significant anti-inflammatory impact by inhibiting NF-kB and NLRP3 inflammasome activation.[9]

FRUIT: AVOCADO

Avocado contains a unique sugar called AV119. Now, you might be thinking sugar is inflammatory, so why would I want sugar? You're right; sugars are inflammatory, but researchers have found that AV119 blocks NF-kB, just like omega-3s do.[10]

DAIRY: GOAT'S MILK

Although A1 dairy is inflammatory, there is one kind of milk—goat's milk—that is anti-inflammatory. One study found that having a little bit of goat cheese ends up cancelling the body's immune system response to lipopoly-saccharides, one type of toxin that leaks out of the gut into the bloodstream because of a weak gut lining.[11] No immune response equals no inflammation.

BEVERAGE: GREEN TEA

If you're not already sipping green tea through-out the day, here's a good reason to start now: Green tea contains the catechin epigal-locatechin gallate (EGCG), shown in multiple studies to neutralize the most inflammatory substances out there, interleukin 8 (IL-8) and tumor necrosis factor-alpha (TNF-α).[12]

FAT: OLIVE OIL

There's a compound in olive oil called oleo-canthal. If you've ever had good, high-quality olive oil, it's what causes that little tingle, or sting, at the back of your throat. You won't get that same sensation with low-quality olive oil because the oleocanthal has been broken down. Researchers have found that oleocanthal has a similar effect to ibuprofen, a nonsteroidal anti-inflammatory drug (NSAID).[13] Like ibuprofen, olive oil prevents the enzyme cyclooxygenase (COX) from doing its job, help-ing control inflammation and ease pain. That's not to say you should just have a shot of olive oil instead of ibuprofen, but over the long term, olive oil is going to attenuate inflammation in a similar fashion.

SPICE: TURMERIC AND GINGER

Why both? Because I can't choose just one.

Traditionally used in Chinese and Indian Ayurvedic medicines to treat arthritis, tur-meric blocks inflammatory cytokines and enzymes, including cyclooxygenase-2 (COX-2), which reduces inflammation. A 2010 clinical trial found that a turmeric supplement with 75 percent curcumin (the main active ingredient in turmeric) provided significant long-term improvement in pain and function in 100 patients with knee osteoarthritis.[14] In a small 2012 pilot study, curcumin was shown to reduce joint pain and swelling in patients with active rheumatoid arthritis better than diclofenac, an NSAID.[15] Turmeric is truly a sus-tainable way to modulate inflammation within your body.

Ginger contains a particularly potent anti-inflammatory compound called gingerol. Gingerol is the reason many sufferers of osteoarthritis or rheumatoid arthritis experi-ence reduced pain levels when they consume

A 2013 study published in *Food & Function* found that adding a little bit of avocado to a beef burger neutralized the inflammatory effects of the burger.[16] Is that a free pass to load up on beef patties as long as you have them with some avo? No. But, it is a compelling example of just how mighty an anti-inflammatory avocados are.

ginger regularly. One study compared the effects of ginger extract to a placebo in 247 patients with osteoarthritis of the knee. The ginger reduced pain and stiffness in knee joints by 40 percent over the placebo![17] Ginger also contains a compound known as 6-shogaol that inhibits the release of swelling-causing chemicals known to cause damage and inflammation to neurons.[18]

Do a Bone Broth "Fast"

I am a huge proponent of bone broth because of how gut healing it is, protecting and supporting the gut mucosal lining, balancing the gut microbiota, and improving gut motility. I use bone broth "fasts" all the time for an intense bout of restoration.

I say "fast" because bone broth is not fasting friendly. If you're eating bone broth, you are not, technically, in a fasting state—too many calories; too much of a metabolic response. I use the term to indicate periods of time, anywhere from sixteen to twenty-four-plus hours, where I follow all the other fasting window guidelines but add bone broth. A bone broth fast once every week or two will help your gut a lot.

SUPPORT YOUR LIVER

The liver filters everything that enters the body—from food and alcohol to medicine and toxins. It determines which nutrients to keep and which chemicals to break down into less harmful forms and remove. It also manages blood sugar levels, metabolizes and stores fats, and regulates sex, thyroid, and other hormones, among roughly 500 essential tasks. When the liver becomes damaged or so overwhelmed it can't do its jobs efficiently or effectively, we've got serious troubles, including inflammation.

Reduce Your Toxic Load

The 80,000 toxins present everywhere in our modern world can significantly stress the liver.[19] They enter our bodies through our mouths, noses, and skin. The more the liver has to focus on filtering them out, the less capacity the liver has to do everything else. Toxins build up in our bodies over time, lodging, especially, in fat tissue. This is why going organic is important—but there's still much more we can do to limit the toxins entering our bodies (it's nearly impossible to eliminate them completely).

CHOOSE NATURAL HOUSEHOLD CLEANING AND PERSONAL CARE PRODUCTS

According to the Environmental Protection Agency (EPA), Americans spend an average of 90 percent of their time indoors, where the air is two to five times more polluted than outside.[20] A major reason for the pollution? Toxic household cleaners that end up on our skin and in the air every time we use them. As with packaged foods, products with a long list of ingredients you can't pronounce are best avoided. In some cases, you may find it cheaper, easier, and more satisfying to use homemade products.

Conventional colognes and perfumes, hair products, lotions, makeup, skin creams, soaps, toothpastes, and anything else in your bathroom cabinet are filled with artificial fragrances and colors and other chemicals. Go with all-natural options or make your own.

Toxins to look out for include:

→ Bisphenol-A (BPA): widely used in plastics and packaging

→ Glycol ethers: including 2-butoxyethanol, ethylene glycol, polyethylene glycol, and propylene glycol, found in cosmetics, degreasers, medications, sunscreens, and water-based paints

→ Parabens: preservatives used in many personal care products

→ Phthalates: chemicals added to plastics to soften them and or personal care products, such as aftershave lotions, hairspray, and shampoos, to "gel" ingredients

→ Triclosan: an antibacterial and antifungal agent often found in toothpaste, soaps, and detergents

FILTER DRINKING WATER

According to the Environmental Working Group (EWG), roughly 85 percent of us drink tap water that contains more than 300 contaminants—more than half of which are not regulated by the EPA.[21] Instead of turning to bottled water, opt for individual filtration units for each of your taps. If you can afford it, add one to your shower (remember, toxins enter through the skin, too) or install a whole-house system.

Test for MTHFR Gene Variants

The MTHFR gene is crucial for a process called methylation, which regulates at least 200 functions in your body, including antioxidant production, cell repair, and immune response. If you have an MTHFR gene variant, you may have trouble metabolizing B vitamins or making enough of the master antioxidant glutathione, both essential for liver detoxification. Genetic testing can determine whether you have a variant. If you do have a variant, work with a trained practitioner to adjust your diet, supplementation, and lifestyle to best support you. Keep in mind, these variants are common. It's estimated that about 40 percent of Americans have at least one.[22]

GO FOR GARLIC

Garlic is rich in a variety of active compounds that support a healthy liver, so add as much to your food as possible.[23] When chopped, crushed, or minced, the alliin in garlic converts to allicin, a potent antioxidant. Selenium increases the action of antioxidants, aiding the liver in its detoxification role. Arginine, an amino acid important for relaxing the blood vessels, eases blood pressure in the liver. High amounts of vitamin B_6 lowers homocysteine, an inflammatory amino acid produced when proteins are broken down, thus easing inflammation within the liver. Garlic can also reduce total serum and LDL cholesterol, the "bad" cholesterol that can damage the liver.[24]

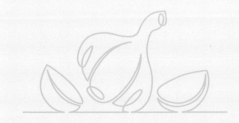

Persistent pathogens, such as viruses, parasites, mold, and bacteria, are an often-overlooked yet persistent source of chronic inflammation.[25] Although active infections cause symptoms that are obvious, as the infectious agent rapidly multiplies, latent infections hide, inactive and dormant in your cells, waiting for the perfect opportunity to re-emerge. Stress, injury, illness, or surgery can cause an infection to roar back to life, firing up your immune system and igniting inflammation.

Common Infectious Agents

- *Borrelia burgdorferi*, the bacteria that causes Lyme disease

- Epstein-Barr virus (EBV), the virus that causes mono

- *Helicobacter pylori* (H. pylori), a bacteria that lives in the digestive tract

- Herpes simplex virus (HSV), which causes genital and/or oral sores

- Mold, a nonscientific term for many types of fungi that cause infections

- Parasites, organisms that live on or in a host organism and get their food from or at the expense of their host; malaria is a well-known parasitic infection, but there are many others including trichomoniasis, a common sexually transmitted disease, and giardiasis, one of the most frequent causes of water-borne disease in the United States

- Varicella-zoster virus (VZV), causes chickenpox and shingles

If you have previously suffered from one of these infections or have troubling, yet undiagnosed, symptoms, discuss this with your health care provider and get tested to rule infection out or begin treatment.

TRY THESE SUPPLEMENTS

The following supplements reduce inflammation in the body and lessen the pain that may accompany it.

Serrapeptase

Take during your eating window. Serrapeptase, an enzyme derived from the intestine of the Japanese silkworm, has been shown to break down nonliving protein tissue (fibrin) that can clog arteries and increase inflammation. And, what's really interesting is, serrapeptase can actually reduce pain and target areas of inflammation by binding to the macroglobulin inside the blood plasma and protecting itself from your immune system to be allowed to do its work. It's a powerful painkiller and anti-inflammatory all in one.

In one study comparing three groups of patients after upper ankle surgery relating to a rupture of the lateral ligament, the group given serrapeptase not only had an instant reduction in pain that was very dramatic, but they also had a 50 percent reduction in inflammation three days postoperative compared to the other two groups.[26] I never thought I'd be adding a funky little enzyme from the intestine of a silkworm to my diet regimen, but the clinical science is no joke.

Glutathione

Take during your eating window. Often referred to as the mother of all antioxidants because it's found in virtually every cell of the human body, glutathione is composed of three amino acids: cysteine, glutamate, and glycine. The highest concentration of glutathione is in the liver, making it a critical component in the body's detoxification process. Glutathione is also an essential component of the body's natural defense system, vitally important in the modulation of the immune system's response. Glutathione is necessary for the creation of white blood cells, the body's first-line infection fighters, and by instructing them, influences the rise and fall of inflammation.[27] Bacteria, certain medications, heavy metal toxicity, radiation, viruses, and even the normal aging process can all cause highly inflammatory free-radical damage to healthy cells and deplete glutathione, tasked with protecting cells and tissues from free-radical harm.[28] Glutathione depletion has been associated with reduced immune function and increased vulnerability to infection due to the liver's reduced ability to detoxify the body. Rebalancing glutathione reduces chronic inflammation on several fronts.[29]

EXERCISE

Exercise triggers robust amounts of inflammation. Working out can cause muscle fibers to tear and muscle cells to break apart. After the workout, our bodies repair the damage we've caused and regrow our muscles even stronger. Any soreness you feel after working out is a sign that damage has been done and your immune system has kicked in to fix it.

Researchers have found that exercise upregulates interleukin 6, or IL-6, a complex protein that has both pro-inflammatory and anti-inflammatory properties. Post-exercise, IL-6 aids recovery by suppressing the inflammatory tumor necrosis factor-alpha (TNF-α). The longer the workout, the more interleukin 6 that's released. For example, after a thirty-minute workout, IL-6 levels may increase fivefold; after a marathon, they may skyrocket by a factor of 100—*and* the more TNF-α that's released.[30] This is why proper recovery, including replacing lost fluids, prioritizing high-quality protein, supplementing adequately, and getting enough rest, is important. Without it, we risk teetering over the inflammation edge where the amount of IL-6 is no longer enough to combat the TNF-α.

On the other hand, quell too much inflammation and you don't get stronger muscles from the rebuild. With exercise and inflammation, it's all about checks and balances.

So, besides proper recovery, how can we strike the right balance and take advantage of the anti-inflammatory benefits of exercise?

Exercise Regularly

Chronic exercise, repeated bouts of exercise over the long term, will give you the anti-inflammatory effect. Yes, acute exercise, or a single routine, will increase anti-inflammatory markers, but chances are, the corresponding inflammatory response within the body will be too high for the body to fully cope with it.[31]

Lose Fat, Especially Belly Fat

Body fat, especially abdominal fat, is very inflammatory. Studies have found that regular exercise increases levels of interleukin 15 (IL-15), a protein that prevents the buildup of belly fat.[32] The leaner you are, the less inflammation you are likely to have. You'll also be in better shape to perform at a higher level and improve your anti-inflammatory response overall.[33]

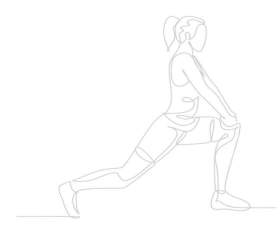

Yoga, with its stress-reducing qualities, may help turn down inflammation in the body. In one study, participants who did yoga for one hour, six days a week, for three months, showed significant decreases in inflammatory markers, such as TNF-α and IL-6, compared to the control group who continued with their usual daily activities but did not do yoga.[34] Maintaining a regular yoga practice brings benefits. In another study, healthy women who regularly practiced hatha yoga were shown to have lower levels of IL-6, the inflammatory marker, overall, and 41 percent less after a task designed to raise their stress levels compared to novice yoga practitioners.[35]

TRY RED LIGHT THERAPY

I've been using red light therapy, also known as photobiomodulation, for a long time. It started as something only biohacking nerds tried because they knew about some of the esoteric science behind it but, over time, it's grown more popular. Research is expanding, too, revealing how our cells are receptive to different kinds of light that can initiate a variety of positive cascades and chain reactions within our bodies.

Red light therapy works by exposing the body to low-wavelength red light, which penetrates the skin and hits the cells, where it is absorbed and used by the mitochondria to produce more energy.[36] When cells are exposed to red light, we see a huge reduction in reactive oxygen species, which means we create less cellular waste, or we produce more energy with less waste. In addition, red light therapy improves nitric oxide activity within the body, which results in increased blood flow.

All of this adds up to red light therapy having a significant anti-inflammatory effect on the body, limiting the inflammatory response, and lowering oxidative damage by reducing inflammatory cytokines, such as TNF-α and interleukin 6 (IL-6).[37]

Many day spas, wellness centers, and dermatology offices offer red light therapy, and red light lamps and therapy devices can be purchased for home use.

LET'S BREAK IT DOWN

- Extend your fasting length a few times every couple of months for a powerful anti-inflammatory reboot.

- Support your gut by ditching inflammatory foods, prioritizing inflammation-fighting foods, and doing bone broth "fasts" to prevent leaky gut.

- Eliminate toxic household and personal care products and filter your water to reduce your toxic load and help your liver perform the more than 500 functions it's responsible for efficiently.

- Try supplements, such as serrapeptase and glutathione, for help rebalancing inflammation.

- Work out regularly to take advantage of exercise's anti-inflammatory benefits and add red light therapy to reduce oxidative damage.

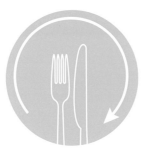

CHAPTER 10

Enhance Your Sleep

I don't sleep well. Like many of you, I have a hard time sleeping because my mind is going all the time. So, I know getting good sleep isn't easy. Add a grinding schedule, children, pets, and noisy neighbors and it can seem impossible—but, it really isn't, and quality sleep is too important to ignore. Poor sleep won't just leave you dragging every day, struggling to maintain a healthy lifestyle, it will also steamroll your health as well as the results you're hoping to achieve with intermittent fasting. Making the extra effort to stop sabotaging my sleep and upgrading its quality has yielded significant dividends, mentally and physically, and it can do the same for you.

SLEEP MATTERS

Deep, restorative sleep is required for a sharp mind, strong body, and weight loss. The brain and body change during sleep, slowing down and focusing on repair and renewal. Muscle repair, protein synthesis, and tissue growth occur during sleep. The brain consolidates new information, converting short-term memories into long-term ones, and clears out the garbage, erasing unnecessary information and removing actual toxic waste, including the harmful beta-amyloid protein linked to brain deterioration.[1] Think of sleep as the essential biological process it is, rather than an inconvenience or "nice" to have if you can get it. Because if you're not getting it, you risk undoing all the results you're working to achieve with intermittent fasting and you will definitely struggle to take those results to the next level.

Talking about sleep can be boring, but the effect poor sleep has on us is truly eye-opening. It can wreck us by promoting:

→ **Weight gain.** We see it all the time. The moment someone starts losing sleep, they start packing on the pounds. Poor sleep dysregulates your hunger hormones, insulin, leptin, and ghrelin, making it easy to pack on the fat. Researchers tracked 1,000 subjects who were getting less than 5 hours of sleep per night. They found a 16 percent decrease in leptin, the satiety hormone that tells your brain you have enough fuel (fat) on hand and can rev up your metabolism to burn it, and a 15 percent increase in ghrelin, a hunger hormone.[2] Those changes alone are the perfect recipe for weight gain.

Another study confirmed the link between sleep and snacking. It found that participants who slept for 4½ hours per night for 4 nights had an increase in 2-arachidonoylglycerol (2-AG), an endocannabinoid involved in modulating hunger and food intake, compared to those who slept for 8½ hours each night.

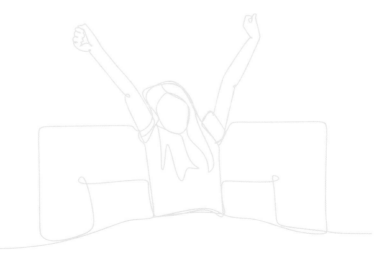

Higher levels of 2-AG activate what I'll call the munchy pathway, significantly increased cravings, the amount of food eaten, and the satisfaction gained from eating. Bring on the munchies, when even cruddy food tastes good, and you're more likely to overindulge in it.[3] Tied to this is the finding that when you are sleep deprived, your reward-seeking behavior changes. You get more stimulated from the reward standpoint of food than you ordinarily would, heightening your response to food in a way that can promote binge eating and food addiction.[4]

→ **Inflammation.** Sleep loss is a major driver of inflammation, upregulating inflammatory cytokines such as tumor necrosis factor-alpha and interleukin 6 (IL-6).[5] Unfortunately, research suggests it takes only one night of bad sleep for you to feel a negative effect. A 2008 study found that one single night of partial sleep resulted in significantly higher levels of nuclear factor-kB (NF-kB), a transcription factor that plays a critical role in triggering inflammation throughout the body. A very important point to note: This increase was only found in female subjects, suggesting poor sleep affects women differently than men and, perhaps, more intensely regarding inflammation.[6] It's an area in need of more study. And, while the immune system is hiking levels of tissue-damaging cytokines, it's downregulating the protective cytokines and antibodies needed to fight infection, making you more vulnerable to sickness.[7]

One organ that takes a negative hit from a lack of sleep—and one we really want to support to control inflammation and weight gain—is the liver. During sleep, the body repairs and renews its cells. Lack of sleep interferes with the liver's ability to do that, straining its ability to function properly when you're awake. Researchers have determined that sleep deprivation can cause oxidative stress to the liver, causing fat to be processed less efficiently and, therefore, allowed to accumulate.[8]

→ **Dysregulated blood glucose and lower insulin sensitivity.** We want to make our bodies more sensitive to insulin and able to use glucose more efficiently, and a lack of sleep does exactly the opposite. One study found significant reductions in insulin sensitivity after one week of sleeping for five hours each night.[9] This is likely linked to the increase in cortisol associated with lack of sleep. The body perceives sleep deprivation as a threat, so cortisol kicks in, which suppresses insulin, flooding the bloodstream with glucose so we have all the energy we need to fight or flee the perceived danger. That danger never really goes away, and chronically elevated cortisol causes blood glucose to remain high and makes cells more resistant to insulin.

Okay, you're sold on sleep. Well, what does good sleep look like anyway? First off, not everyone needs the same amount of shut-eye. The National Sleep Foundation advises adults ages 26 to 64 to get 7 to 9 hours' sleep, whereas adults 65 years and older should aim for 7 to 8 hours of sleep.[10] Seven to nine hours may be optimal for most people, but the amount of sleep you need is highly individual and dependent on your specific biology.[11] So, don't stress out if you need a little less or a little more. What really matters is the quality of your sleep. You're getting good quality sleep if you:

→ Sleep for at least 85 percent of the total time you are in bed

→ Fall asleep in 30 minutes or fewer

→ Wake up no more than once per night

→ Can go back to sleep within 20 minutes if you wake up in the middle of the night

→ Wake rested and energized in the morning[12]

Whether you're simply not getting enough quality sleep, or you are looking for ways to get more benefit from less sleep, you'll find that by implementing the following suggestions you'll get into deeper sleep more quickly. Supercharge your sleep and you supercharge your results. Let's get to it.

TOP TACTIC

GET ENOUGH VITAMIN D

Low levels of vitamin D are associated with sleep problems, including insufficient sleep (less than five hours per night), difficulty falling asleep, restless or fragmented sleep, and overall poor sleep quality.[13] Many studies also link vitamin D deficiency to sleep apnea, perhaps because low vitamin D has been shown to increase inflammation of the nose and throat.[14]

THE ESSENTIALS

Improving sleep isn't magic, but it is a science, and there are some basic research-backed approaches to help you stop sleeping like garbage. We want to match what's happening externally with what's happening internally.

Sleep in Alignment with Your Circadian Rhythm

Many mental and physical systems in your body run according to a circadian rhythm, a twenty-four-hour cycle.[15] (The term *circadian* comes from the Latin phrase "circa diem," meaning "around a day.") Hormones rise and ebb throughout the day, regulating everything from sleep and hunger to alertness, body temperature, metabolism, and mood. Just about every tissue and organ has a clock, and these individual clocks are controlled by the master clock located in the suprachiasmatic nucleus (SCN) part of the brain. Throughout the day, the SCN instructs and coordinates the activities of all the other body clocks. We tend to overlook one very important fact about the SCN: It is highly sensitive to light. (Light isn't the only influencer, but it is the most powerful one, and it is the reason our brains time the performance of certain functions to day and night.)

When it comes to sleep, darkness triggers the SCN to tell the cells to slow down and prepare for rest.[16] The hormone melatonin level rises to relax the body and get it ready for sleep. Melatonin levels peak between 2 a.m. and 4 a.m., then taper off. As morning comes and light increases, the SCN signals cortisol to rise, which promotes wakefulness. To the SCN, night means restorative mode and day means active mode. When we're in sync with our circadian rhythm, we sleep better and are energized during the day. When we're out of sync, we find it difficult to fall or stay asleep and experience a cascade of hormone imbalances due to an out of whack SCN. This is why poor sleep affects so many aspects of health.

Syncing is easier said than done, I know. Modern life is full of nonstop demands coming at us at all hours, encouraging us to be on high alert, checking devices, staying up, and eating way past when darkness falls, all of which makes it tough to sync and stay synced with our circadian rhythm. Then, there are those of us who work the night shift and are chronically at odds with evening hours and the restoration mode they should bring. (Check out the box on page 174 with suggestions for ways to support your body and minimize the negative impact of always being out of sync.) But, living in line with your natural clocks and rhythms will have a profoundly positive effect on your metabolism and energy levels, helping you feel more awake and alive and better able to make good choices and work out at the intensity level you want.

Use Fasting to Restore Sleep Patterns

New evidence suggests you can use intermittent fasting to help get you into alignment and restore your sleep patterns in a short time. Researchers divided participants into two groups. One group fasted for eighteen hours with an eating window between 8 a.m. and 2 p.m. *Note that timing.* The second group ate between 8 a.m. and 8 p.m., a twelve-hour eating window, which is still very good compared to how nonstop most of the world eats. Results indicated that the time-restricted eating group, the group that ate in the morning, had a huge increase in the expression of clock genes, genes that regulate the circadian rhythm. The researchers also found an increase in SIRT1 genes, which are associated with longevity, but it turns out they can also act as clock genes and help us reset our circadian rhythm. By compressing the eating window to four hours in the morning, participants experienced circadian synchronization in just four days.[17]

Now, I don't recommend fasting for eighteen hours for four days in a row. But this research suggests that fasting with a morning eating window is one tool in our good sleep tool kit worth trying to get back in alignment.

Can You Pay Back Your Weekly Sleep Debt on the Weekend?

Sleep debt is the difference between the amount of sleep you should be getting and the amount you actually get. The bad news: That debt grows every time you cut your sleeping time short. The good news: Sleep debt can be repaid, but it doesn't happen after just one extended sleep over a weekend. One study found that make-up sleep on the weekends erased some of the deficits, such as soaring inflammation, associated with not sleeping enough the previous week—but attention, cognitive function, and focus took longer to rebound.[18] Instead of sleeping for twelve hours straight, add an extra fifteen to twenty minutes of sleep each night (an hour if you can manage it!) to catch up over time. If you're chronically sleep deprived, it may take you a few months to get back to baseline.

Practice Good Sleep Habits

The thing is, you need to do most, if not all, of these suggestions to get results. Your body needs the cumulative impact of all of these strategies to align with your circadian rhythm. Doing just one or two isn't going to result in a whole lot of good. That said, creating new habits can be challenging. Start by introducing one or two each week until you've got them all covered.

DURING THE DAY

→ **First thing in the morning, get light.** If the weather and temperature are conducive, stand outside in natural light for fifteen to thirty minutes, so your brain can recognize it's morning and time to get the body going. If you don't have the right conditions to go outside, use red light therapy bulbs to initiate the same response.

→ **Get into a morning routine.** For example, wake up (at about the same time each morning), get light, exercise, then eat. Keeping to a regular schedule helps your SCN lock in that it is daytime.

→ **Be outside as much as possible.** We're typically inside all day, or most of the day, so try to get some sun during the day. Take a quick walk after lunch, for example, to reinforce daytime as active time.

IN THE EVENING

→ **Aim for a consistent bedtime.** A regular sleep time cues your body to anticipate rest at the same time each evening and prep effectively.

→ **Don't eat right before bedtime.** Less light means the SCN signals cells to shut things down, including digestion. Eating after dark, and especially late in the evening, runs counter to everything your body is trying to accomplish. You might feel good initially, but eventually your blood sugar will fall, and when your blood sugar falls, cortisol is released to bring it back up. That middle-of-the-night fight-or-flight hormone surge is going to wake you up and bump you out of restorative sleep. Instead, get in alignment by having your last meal before dark, which is good for your sleep and good for your scale.

A recent study looked at 82 people who ate the same reduced-calorie diet. One group had their last meal between 7 p.m. and 7:30 p.m., and the other group ate their last meal between 10:30 p.m. and 11 p.m. Both groups lost weight—no real surprise here, as both groups were intentionally eating fewer calories—but the group that ate their last meal between 7 and 7:30 lost almost 5 pounds (2.25 kg) more and had significantly better insulin response and fasting glucose, cholesterol, and triglyceride levels.[19] A calorie is more than a calorie, depending on when it's consumed.

SLEEP TIPS FOR NIGHT SHIFT WORKERS

Try to get your body into a pattern so it comes to expect sleeping and waking at regular times. Even if your schedule is wildly erratic, you can use these tips to cue your body that it's time for rest and get to sleep faster.

1. **Use light therapy.** Manipulate light to trigger the release of melatonin and promote sleep. It's 11 a.m. and you're just getting home. Draw the curtains and dim the lights. Now, it's midnight and you're getting up. Turn up the bright lights.

2. **Eat some carbs before bed.** Carbohydrates promote the hormone serotonin, which signals melatonin and sleep.[20] You don't need much, just 0.25 gram of carbohydrates per pound of body weight, within three to four hours of going to bed.

3. **Take a hot bath before bed.** Sure, it's relaxing, but a hot bath also elevates your core body temperature. When you get out of the bath, your body starts to cool down, releasing melatonin and promoting sleep.

→ **Limit caffeine and alcohol before bedtime.** Caffeine blocks adenosine, a chemical in the brain that accumulates throughout the day making us sleepier as the day goes on. Caffeine reduces our sleepiness, and when taken too close to bed, defies our natural circadian rhythm and makes it tough to get to sleep. I suggest stopping caffeine in the afternoon, a good six hours before bed.

A glass of wine after dinner may seem to help you sleep because it makes you drowsy, but alcohol is sugar, and once your blood sugar crashes, cortisol spikes, waking you up in the middle of the night and sabotaging restorative sleep. And, that drowsy feeling? Alcohol jacks up GABA to the point where you feel relaxed, but you don't actually get into the REM phase of sleep or stay in the REM phase long enough. REM is an important part of the sleep cycle associated with benefits to learning, memory, and mood. Several studies confirm that alcohol before bed reduces the amount of REM sleep and extends the amount of time it takes to enter REM, meaning the overall amount of REM sleep is far less. That's a double whammy if you're already challenged to get enough hours snoozing.[21]

➜ **Avoid vigorous exercise within an hour of bedtime.** Exercise increases your heart rate and core body temperature, two things we want to be lowering in order to sleep. Studies have shown that nonvigorous exercise, such as Tai Chi, walking, or yoga, is fine, but vigorous exercise, such as weight training, intervals, and high-intensity cardio, will make it tough to get to sleep and stay asleep.[22]

➜ **Power down before bedtime.** Artificial light in the evening, especially the blue light emitted from electronic devices, sends the wrong signals to our brains, stopping melatonin production. Limit all artificial light in the evening (dimmer switches are a good way to do this) and turn away from electronic devices such as computers, phones, and televisions at least an hour before bed.

If you must be connected at night, use blue light–blocking glasses. They may not be the most fashion-forward eyewear, but studies demonstrate that wearing blue light–blocking glasses has a hugely helpful effect on your circadian rhythm. In one study, researchers exposed one set of subjects to blue light whereas another set received blue light–blocking glasses. Well, lo and behold, the group that had the blue light–blocking glasses experienced significantly improved sleep quality and mood.[23] So, they slept better and felt better. Pretty powerful stuff.

➜ **Keep it dark.** Light is sleep's kryptonite. Block out the light and keep your room super dark for deeper sleep. Use blackout blinds to prevent outside light from creeping in but don't forget to remove or cover devices that give off light, too. Think an alarm clock. Even easier: Wear a sleep mask.

➜ **Keep it cool.** We sleep best when the thermostat is set between 60°F and 67°F (15.5°C and 19.4°C) because our core body temperature drops as part of the process that helps us fall asleep and keeps us there throughout the night.[24] When darkness falls and melatonin is released, your core temperature starts to lower. The blood vessels at peripheral sites around your body dilate, so hot blood gets shunted away from your core and dissipates through your arms, hands, legs, feet, and head. Your core cools and its temperature keeps dropping until early morning when it starts to rise again as the body wakes up. A bedroom that's too hot is uncomfortable, makes it tough to get to sleep, and might cause you to wake in the middle of the night.[25] Think about it. Do you sleep better with an air conditioner or fan running or a window open? Yeah, me too.

In addition to keeping your sleeping environment as cool as possible, opt for breathable moisture-wicking fabrics (linen, cotton) for your bedding to keep your body temperature in the comfort zone. I also recommend a cooling mattress pad, especially one that allows you to adjust the temperature. Set it so the temperature rises slowly and wakes you naturally in the morning. I've noticed a big difference in my sleep with one—I stay asleep longer and I fall asleep more easily.

→ **Get checked out.** Chronic daytime sleepiness and low energy, or symptoms such as snoring, choking, or gasping sounds and jerking leg movements, may be signs of a sleep disorder such as sleep apnea (temporary lapses in breathing), restless leg syndrome, or another health condition. Don't ignore the signs—or your sleeping partner's complaints—and speak to your health care provider about them.

Essential Sleep Habits

- First thing in the morning, get light.

- Get into a morning routine.

- Be outside as much as possible.

- Aim for a consistent bedtime.

- Don't eat right before bedtime.

- Limit caffeine and alcohol before bedtime.

- Avoid vigorous exercise within an hour of bedtime.

- Power down before bedtime.

- Keep your bedroom dark and cool.

- Get checked out. Don't ignore snoring or other signs of a potential sleep disorder.

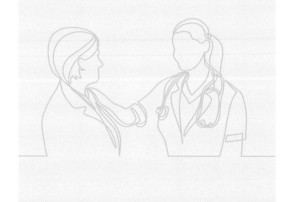

THE ENHANCEMENTS

Try these enhancements *after* you've nailed the essentials but need a little extra help to get back in alignment with your circadian rhythm or want to upgrade your sleep quality.

Strategic Supplementation with Melatonin

Okay to take during your fasting window. To be clear: I am not a fan of taking melatonin as a sleep aid regularly because, by giving your body this hormone every evening, your body adjusts to having melatonin supplied rather than to manufacturing it. The neurons in the SCN have receptors for melatonin, and if we take a supplement, surging the amount of melatonin in our bodies, we essentially burn out those receptors, leaving us dependent on supplementation.[26] That's not what we want. And, disrupting melatonin disrupts other hormones, throwing off your entire endocrine system. It's not worth it.

However, studies support that the occasional, or even one-off, use of melatonin to support a new pattern can be very effective at restoring circadian rhythm.[27] Take 1 mg of melatonin about an hour before eating your last meal of the day to give your body time to digest the meal and wind down. Then, keep to this eating and sleeping schedule *without the melatonin*. Remember, the melatonin supplement is only to support your new sleep-supporting lifestyle habits. Use melatonin one time, or certainly no more than once every three weeks, then allow your body to restore its rhythm naturally.

Supplement with Magnesium

Okay to take during your fasting window. Magnesium promotes calm by activating the parasympathetic nervous system, responsible for the relaxation response, which helps us chill out.[28] One of the most interesting things about magnesium when it comes to sleep is that it blocks cortisol in the brain. By preventing cortisol from hitting the brain, magnesium stops the brain from sending signals that keep you anxious, wired, and unable to sleep. On the other hand, it increases gamma-aminobutyric acid (GABA), a neurotransmitter that lowers nerve activity, exactly what we want to have elevated when we're falling asleep.[29] Another awesome thing about magnesium is that it regulates the production of melatonin.[30] More magnesium correlates with more melatonin. By supporting the natural production of melatonin, we avoid the dependency trap of taking the hormone directly.

Supplement with L-theanine

Okay to take during your fasting window. L-theanine promotes sleep by enhancing the production of GABA, serotonin, which converts to melatonin, and alpha waves in the brain, an indicator of relaxation.[31] In one study, healthy adults given L-theanine for four weeks fell asleep more quickly and had fewer sleep disturbances than those given a placebo.[32]

Supplement with Glycine

Only take during your eating window. Glycine, an amino acid, promotes a cooling effect in the body by decreasing blood flow and temperature to subcutaneous areas. When we cool the body, there is an increase in melatonin. Supplementing with glycine has been shown to improve sleep quality, shorten the length of time it takes to fall asleep, lessen daytime sleepiness, and improve cognitive function. [33]

Coffee Nap Hack

What? After everything about reining in caffeine before sleep—how can it be a part of a sleep hack? Hold tight. Adenosine (the central building block of ATP, the main energy currency) is a neurochemical that helps us sleep. It's generated during waking hours and decreases during sleep. The longer we are awake, the more adenosine that accumulates, and the more we are driven to sleep. Caffeine works by binding and blocking adenosine receptors. The caffeine in a cup of coffee prevents adenosine from hitting the receptors and making us tired. By drinking a caffeinated beverage, we blunt the tiredness.

So, here's how the coffee nap hack works: Have a cup of coffee, then immediately take a fifteen- to thirty-minute nap. Hit that nap hard! Because while you're napping, the extra adenosine gets let into the receptors. All the adenosine building up and up and up and making you tired hits the receptors and is relieved. Now the caffeine comes into play and blocks any more adenosine from accessing the receptors. You've killed two birds with

TOP TACTIC

RED LIGHT THERAPY FOR GOOD SLEEP

I tried red light therapy when I was really struggling with a brutal bout of insomnia. It turned things around for me completely. If we spent a lot of time outdoors in the morning and during the day, we'd get plenty of red light, which signals to the SCN that our bodies should be up and in active mode. But we don't. We spend most of our time indoors, not getting enough red light. Red light therapy amplifies the signaling to the SCN, helping align with your circadian rhythm and, ultimately, enhancing your ability to get to sleep later on.

Scientists found that study participants who did just thirty minutes of red light therapy for fourteen days produced almost double the amount of melatonin as those who did not.[34] Just two weeks is all it took to see a benefit, and that fact rings true to my experience.

ENHANCE YOUR SLEEP

Supplement with:

✓ Melatonin (*strategically*)

✓ Magnesium

✓ L-theanine

✓ Glycine

Try a coffee nap hack:

Keep it quiet

one hack: You have drained away excess adenosine, leaving you feeling refreshed, and you've blocked the receptors with caffeine, so no more adenosine can gain entry. You can have caffeine without crashing later and get a very restorative effect in a brief period of time. In one study, consuming caffeine followed by a fifteen-minute power nap increased overall wakefulness by 91 percent—and subjects slept normally later on.[35] By adding the nap, they didn't just have the usual all-too-brief caffeine lift, they fixed their tiredness issue.

Keep It Quiet

Blocking light with blackout curtains or a sleep mask is a great start to limiting sensory deprivation, but cancelling noise will help even more. If you have noise-cancelling headphones, try sleeping with them on. Soundproof curtains that muffle noise are another option. Add a draft stopper at the base of your door to prevent sound leaking in that way. Besides heat and light, noise is what most commonly wakes people up. Keep it *quiet*. What about a white noise machine or app? Obviously, they won't make your room quiet, but they can drown out sounds that might otherwise wake you up, such as a car horn.

LET'S BREAK IT DOWN

- Poor sleep steamrolls your health as well as the results you're hoping to achieve with intermittent fasting by contributing to inflammation, insulin resistance, and weight gain—among other serious short- and long-term health consequences.

- You can achieve better quality sleep through several simple daily circadian rhythm–supporting habits.

- It's the cumulative effect of these sleep habits, not one-offs occasionally, that will get you into a deeper sleep. Commit to consistently incorporating one or two at a time as part of your lifestyle to see real results.

- Use additional strategies, such as supplementation and the coffee nap hack, for extra support syncing with your circadian rhythm, or to get more out of your sleep.

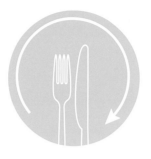

CHAPTER 11

Additional Strategies for Women

Throughout the book, I've pointed out specific recommendations for women to support your unique biology. I'd like to give some extra attention, though, to two common issues women struggle with that can cause a cascade of hormonal imbalances and stall fat burning and weight loss and offer strategies for restoring balance.

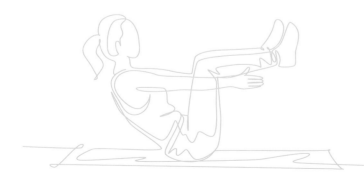

These are:

✓ Estrogen dominance

✓ Symptoms of low thyroid function

By maintaining good hormone alignment, you'll feel amazing, be your best self, and reap the rewards of all the hard work you're doing to optimize your health and wellness through intermittent fasting.

ESTROGEN DOMINANCE

Estrogen dominance occurs when your body has too much estrogen compared to its counterbalancing hormone, progesterone. It's a lot more common in women of all ages than you may think due to several lifestyle factors, such as high levels of stress and poor gut health, and environmental ones, such as the flood of estrogen-mimicking chemicals in our homes, communities, and foods. The good news is, there's a lot you are already doing to promote good balance.

Estrogen's Role

Estrogen is the primary female sex hormone and an umbrella term for three main types of estrogen:

1. **Estrone (E1):** Responsible for sexual development and function, estrone is considered a weak estrogen and can be converted to another type of estrogen, estradiol (E2), when necessary. Estrone is found in the highest quantities in menopausal women.

2. **Estradiol (E2):** The most potent of the three estrogens, estradiol takes the lead during the menstrual cycle, causing the maturation and release of the egg.

3. **Estriol (E3):** The primary estrogen present during pregnancy, estriol is released in massive quantities by the placenta.

The ovaries are the main source of estrogen in cycling women, though estrogen can also be made by the adrenals, triangular-shaped glands perched on top of both kidneys, and fat tissue. After menopause, when menstruation has ceased, estrogen comes mainly from fat tissue.

The fact that estrogen is responsible for the growth and maintenance of the reproductive system and secondary sex characteristics and regulation of the menstrual cycle likely sounds familiar. What may sound new is, there are estrogen receptors throughout your body.[1] Just about every organ—from your brain to your bladder, bones, and heart—relies on estrogen to function well. This is one reason an estrogen imbalance can sabotage your efforts at fat loss so effectively and make you feel miserable.

Symptoms

When estrogen levels are off kilter, you can feel it in lots of ways. Some of the most common symptoms of estrogen dominance include:

→ Bloating

→ Fatigue

→ Fibrocystic breasts, breast swelling and tenderness

→ Irritability, mood swings

→ Painful PMS

→ Period problems, such as irregular and heavy bleeding

→ Uterine fibroids

→ Weight gain, especially around the hips, belly, and thighs

Causes

Too much estrogen is just one reason for estrogen dominance. To really understand what's going on, we have to look deeper at all the ways estrogen can become imbalanced, including poor estrogen metabolism and clearance.

→ **Too much estradiol (E2).** This powerful estrogen is beneficial in the right doses, but too much of it leads to body-wide symptoms.

→ **Low progesterone.** The hormone progesterone is tasked with thickening the uterine lining to accept an egg after ovulation. It also aids the development of the fetus and prepares the body for labor. Low progesterone makes it difficult to get and stay pregnant. But, like estrogen, progesterone factors into more than fertility. Progesterone also supports brain, heart, nervous system, and thyroid health and stimulates the brain's GABA receptors, producing calming, anti-anxiety effects.[2]

→ **When estrogen and progesterone are in balance, keeping each other in check, things run smoothly.** When it comes to estrogen dominance, too little progesterone means there's not enough to effectively counterbalance the estrogen. Your estrogen levels could be in a normal range, but without enough progesterone to balance the estrogen, you'll experience symptoms of estrogen dominance. Progesterone declines naturally as women enter perimenopause (the transitional period before menopause, the cessation of your period for one year) usually in their late thirties or forties, which is why women are more prone to estrogen dominance during this time.[3]

→ **A poor breakdown of estrogen into too many "bad" metabolites.** The liver is responsible for breaking down used estrogen into smaller forms, called metabolites, and processing them, so they can, ultimately, be excreted from the body through the colon. Some metabolites are better than others; those called 4-hydroxyestrone and 16-alpha-hydroxyestrone are considered "bad," as too many can be harmful to our body.[4] We want to limit the creation of these metabolites

If you've had your gallbladder removed,
you are more vulnerable to estrogen dominance.
Bile, stored in the gallbladder, helps the liver rid
the body of estrogen metabolites. Without a
gallbladder, you may have more difficulty removing
metabolized estrogen, leading to a buildup and the
symptoms of estrogen dominance.

as much as possible, but an overwhelmed liver may lean on the pathways that create these metabolites too frequently, leading to a buildup of these substances and symptoms of estrogen dominance.

→ **Xenoestrogens.** These manmade chemicals, such as BPA, parabens, and phthalates, mimic the behavior of endogenous estrogens, estrogens made by the body, and throw off your hormonal balance by blocking or binding to estrogen receptors and preventing endogenous estrogen from accessing the cells. This is why they are called endocrine disruptors. They are bad for your liver (see chapter 9), and they are bad for your hormones. And did I mention they hide out in fatty tissues, building up over time? One more reason to clear out these chemicals from your home and lifestyle and limit your exposure as much as possible.

Supporting Estrogen Balance

By intermittent fasting and working to amplify your results by crushing inflammation, you're already promoting good balance in a few ways. Here's how:

→ **Promoting fat loss.** The more fat cells you have, the more estrogen your body creates. But it doesn't stop there. Body fat also stores excess estrogen, including all those xenoestrogens.

TOP TACTIC

PRIORITIZE THE ELIMINATION OF SKINCARE PRODUCTS

Xenoestrogens that enter our bodies through the skin, such as via deodorant, lotion, makeup, shampoo, and sunscreen, are absorbed directly into the bloodstream and tissues throughout your body, bypassing the liver's detoxification process. To help prioritize your detoxing, aim to replace these products with natural options.

→ **Crushing inflammation.** Chronic inflammation strains the gut and liver, directly affecting their ability to detoxify estrogen and estrogen levels. You read that right: Your gut helps break down estrogen, too. Once the liver has done its job breaking down estrogen, it sends the processed estrogen in bile through the gallbladder and into the intestines to be broken down further before it can be excreted. That's when a special group of bacteria, called the estrobolome, take over.[5] If your microbiome is unhealthy and you don't have enough of these bacteria, estrogen can be reactivated and sent right back into your bloodstream instead of being removed from the body, driving estrogen dominance.[6] Keeping estrogen levels in balance requires a healthy gut *and* liver to detoxify estrogen properly.

There a few more ways you can support good balance, including:

→ **Eliminate xenoestrogens.** Clearing toxins from our lives is important, so I can't emphasize it enough. Remember:

- ✓ Avoid plastics (food and beverage storage containers and wrap).

- ✓ Choose organic: Herbicides, insecticides, and pesticides are all sources of xenoestrogens.

- ✓ Filter your water.

- ✓ Get rid of products with fake fragrances, including air fresheners (opt for essential oils instead).

- ✓ Go natural for cleaning and personal care products.

- ✓ Open your windows often.

→ **Eat cruciferous vegetables.** These vegetables provide two powerful compounds that support the liver and healthy estrogen detoxification: diindolylmethane (DIM) and sulforaphane.

DIM is produced when stomach acid breaks down cruciferous vegetables. This compound supports estrogen balance by promoting the breakdown of estrogen into the more beneficial 2-hydroxyestrone metabolites instead of the potentially harmful ones, 4-hydroxyestrone and 16 alpha-hydroxyestrone, and may also lower the potency of the latter.[7] DIM has also been shown to block aromatase, the enzyme that converts testosterone to estrogen, encouraging better balance.[8]

Sulforaphane also aids estrogen detoxification and is a powerful antioxidant and anti-inflammatory.[9]

So, eat plenty of arugula, bok choy, broccoli, broccoli sprouts, Brussels sprouts, cabbage, cauliflower, collard greens, kale, radishes, and Swiss chard, or consider supplementation.

→ **Get plenty of fiber.** Once estrogen travels through the liver and gut, it's time to be rid of it through a bowel movement. Eating enough fiber will help keep you regular and those deactivated estrogens moving out of your body in a timely manner. The United States Department of Agriculture (USDA) recommends 14 grams of fiber per each 1,000 calories of food, so a 2,000-calorie-per-day diet would include a recommended fiber intake of 28 grams.[10] Odds are, you're not getting enough fiber. Both soluble (the kind that dissolves in water, found in asparagus and leeks) and insoluble fiber (the kind that doesn't dissolve in water, found in cruciferous vegetables and sweet potatoes) will help clear metabolized estrogens and maintain good balance, so add fiber-rich vegetables to each meal.

What About Phytoestrogens?

Phytoestrogens are estrogenic compounds naturally found in fruits, legumes, vegetables, and some grains. Soy and flaxseed are two of the most common sources of phytoestrogens.[11] Phytoestrogens work like the estrogen produced by our bodies and are able to bind to estrogen receptors. At first, that sounds like a bad idea, especially if you are estrogen dominant. The last thing your body needs is more estrogen, right? The interesting thing about phytoestrogens is that they are much weaker than the body's estrogen, from 100 to 1,000 times less powerful.[12] They are also adaptogenic, meaning they can help restore balance depending on what your body needs, modulating estrogen levels if they are too high or too low.[13] Some women find that phytoestrogens, such as organic, unprocessed or minimally processed soy (edamame, miso, tamari, tempeh) and flaxseed, bring relief from symptoms of estrogen dominance by preventing more potent estrogens from binding to estrogen receptors instead, whereas others find they make them feel worse.[14] This is where your bio-individuality comes into play and why you'll want to experiment to find out what works best for you.

SYMPTOMS OF LOW THYROID FUNCTION

Many women deal with a thyroid issue, whether they've been diagnosed with one or not. The American Thyroid Association estimates that twenty million Americans currently have some form of thyroid condition, with up to 60 percent of them being undiagnosed.[15] When it comes to women specifically, the ATA projects that one in eight women will develop a thyroid condition during her lifetime, and women are five to eight times more likely to develop one than men.[16]

One of the most common thyroid conditions is hypothyroidism, or an underactive thyroid, where the thyroid gland does not make enough thyroid hormones. The culprit is often Hashimoto's thyroiditis, an autoimmune disease in which an overactive immune system attacks and damages the thyroid gland. Many more women struggle with symptoms of low thyroid function, even if their thyroid gland is in perfectly good shape and producing adequate levels of hormones. That's what often makes diagnosing thyroid-related conditions so challenging.

That said, you don't need a diagnosis to know it's a good idea to support your thyroid and the healthy functioning of thyroid hormones as much as you can.

The Thyroid's Role

For a small gland, the thyroid plays a huge part in how well your body runs. A butterfly-shaped organ located at the base of your neck, the thyroid helps control body temperature, breathing, heart rate, liver function, metabolism, muscle and bone development, menstrual cycle, and much more. There are three main thyroid hormones:

1. **Thyroid-stimulating hormone (TSH):** Produced in the pituitary gland, TSH triggers the production and release of thyroxine and triiodothyronine.

2. **Thyroxine (T4):** This main thyroid hormone is delivered directly into the bloodstream by the thyroid gland. T4 is inactive and can't be used by the body as is, but, rather, needs to be converted into T3, the active form of thyroid hormone, by the gut, kidneys, and liver.

3. **Triiodothyronine (T3):** The active form of thyroid hormone; about 20 percent or T3 is made by the thyroid gland itself, with the rest coming from the conversion of T4.

When everything is working as it should, levels of T4 and T3 modulate the release of TSH. When these levels drop, the pituitary gland sends out TSH to tell the thyroid to start producing more. When T4 and T3 levels return to baseline, the pituitary pulls back on TSH to restore equilibrium. If even one piece of this process goes awry, an underproduction of these hormones or low availability of T3 may result. And, because thyroid hormones have a hand in almost everything your body does, and every human cell has thyroid hormone receptors, you'll feel symptoms of this skewed system across your entire body—from energy and mood to digestive and immune system function.

Symptoms

When thyroid hormone levels are low, or T3 is blocked from entering cells, you may experience these symptoms of low thyroid function:

→ Crushing fatigue
→ Weight gain
→ Brain fog
→ Low body temperature, cold hands and feet
→ Dry skin
→ Dry, thinning hair
→ Muscle weakness, aches, and stiffness
→ Constipation
→ Irregular periods
→ Difficulty getting and staying pregnant[17]

Causes

→ **Estrogen dominance.** Too much estrogen blocks thyroid hormone from locking into thyroid hormone receptors and entering the cells.[18] Too much estrogen also increases the amount of thyroid binding globulin (TBG), which does just what it sounds like, binding thyroid hormone so it can't be used, reducing the overall amount of thyroid hormone available to cells.[19] In both cases, thyroid hormone is unable to get where it's needed.

→ **Stress.** Cortisol inhibits the production of TSH, so the thyroid doesn't get the signal to produce T4 and T3 and hits the brakes on the conversion of T4 to T3.[20]

→ **Autoimmune diseases, such as Hashimoto's thyroiditis.** The immune system mistakes healthy tissue, in this case the thyroid gland, as a threat and attacks it, physically damaging the organ and impairing its ability to function.

→ **Iodine deficiency.** Iodine is essential for the creation of thyroid hormones, and because the body can't produce it, we must consume sufficient amounts of it.

→ **Toxins.** Those endocrine-disrupting toxins strike again, mimicking thyroid hormone and blocking thyroid hormone receptors, or damaging the thyroid gland directly. Toxins also elevate estrogen levels, which contribute to low thyroid function.[21] Some of the top toxin offenders when it comes to the thyroid include:

Perchlorate. This industrial chemical used to make rubber, paint, and batteries collects in groundwater and soil, contaminating drinking water, crops, and animals.[22] It's been shown to significantly lower T4 in women and compete with iodine for uptake in the thyroid, compromising the production of thyroid hormone.[23]

PCBs. Though banned in the United States in 1979, this chemical has staying power in the environment. PCBs come at the thyroid in several ways: diminishing its ability to absorb iodine, reducing T4 levels, and making the gland less responsive to TSH.[24]

Dioxin. This byproduct of pesticide and plastic manufacturing can damage the thyroid even at low levels, lowering T4 and thyroid function.[25]

BPA. BPA locks into thyroid receptors, preventing thyroid hormones from accessing cells.[26]

Phthalates. Found in many personal care products, phthalates inhibit thyroid receptor function.[27]

Triclosan. Added to products because of its antibacterial properties, triclosan is associated with decreased levels of T4.[28]

Heavy metals. Mercury, found in seafood, and aluminum, found in makeup, cookware, and antiperspirants, are bad news for your thyroid. Mercury builds up in the thyroid, undermining the thyroid's ability to uptake iodine and make hormones.[29] Aluminum has been shown to damage the thyroid more directly, weakening its ability to function, while also triggering an autoimmune response in the body and the release of antibodies that may target the thyroid.[30]

Getting Tested

If you suspect you have a thyroid issue, speak with your health care provider about getting tested and monitoring your thyroid hormone levels, especially as you incorporate intermittent fasting into your lifestyle. (If you have been diagnosed with a thyroid condition and are intermittent fasting, be sure to monitor your levels as well.) When you speak with your provider:

1. Ask for a full thyroid panel including TSH, total T4 and T3, free T4 and T3, reverse T3, thyroid peroxidase antibodies (TPO), and thyroglobulin antibodies (TGAB). Testing only TSH or TSH and total T4 levels, standard recommendations, isn't enough to tell the full story of what may be going on in your body.

2. Conventional medical lab ranges of what constitute "normal" vary from lab to lab and are based on a statistical average of people previously tested and who, therefore, have a high probability of already being sick. This situation often leads to people falling into "normal" ranges when they're experiencing symptoms. Know what ranges are being used to assess your results and why.

3. Listen to your body. If you don't feel fine, you don't feel fine no matter what a test says. Advocate for your health—or find another practitioner willing to listen to and work with you.

Supporting Your Thyroid and Thyroid Hormones

By intermittent fasting and working to amplify your results by crushing inflammation, you're already working for your thyroid.

Inflammation is closely associated with autoimmune conditions, so keeping inflammation in check supports a healthy immune system.[31] One area of particular importance is gut health. The thyroid relies on several vitamins and minerals, such as iodine, selenium, vitamins A, B, C, and E, and zinc, to produce and metabolize thyroid hormones. If your GI tract is compromised and you aren't able to absorb these nutrients, your thyroid won't be able to use them—no matter how much nutrient-dense food or supplements you consume. And we can't overlook the microbiome. (Again!) About 20 percent of inactive T4 is converted to active T3 in the gut, and this conversion relies on healthy gut bacteria. If your gut is overrun with "bad" bacteria, you're seriously compromising your thyroid hormone levels.

There a few more ways you can support good balance, including eating foods rich in:

Iodine. Good thyroid function and hormone balance rely on iodine, and seaweed is an excellent source of this important mineral. Including iodine as part of breaking your fast is a good idea, but don't stop there. Find ways to add kelp (and kelp seasonings), hijiki, and wakame throughout your eating window.

Zinc. Zinc is required for thyroid hormone production, and zinc allows the hormone receptors in the body to see and accept the active thyroid hormone (T3) that's floating in the bloodstream.[32] We may have adequate T3 levels, but if we don't have any receptors willing to open the door to let T3 enter, then it's not doing us any good. Shellfish, meat, lentils, and chickpeas are good sources of zinc.

Selenium. The mineral selenium is necessary for the conversion of inactive T4 to active T3.[33] Brazil nuts are the quickest and easiest way to get selenium into your diet. You don't need to eat a lot—just two or three nuts do the trick. Cold-water fish, such as sardines, are also high in selenium.

→ **Avoid toxins.**

I know, *again with the toxins*. Reducing your toxic load could be a game changer for your thyroid, liver, and overall hormone balance. Being aware of what you put on your body as much as you are of what you put inside it will boost your ability to be your best self in every possible way. According to some studies, there are more than 150 household chemicals with the potential to directly affect

TRUE OR FALSE

Cruciferous Vegetables Are Bad for Your Thyroid.

False!
Although cruciferous vegetables do contain goitrogens, a naturally occurring compound that can hinder the thyroid's ability to take up iodine, you would have to eat an excessive, unrealistic amount of these vegetables over an extended period of time for interference to occur. [34]

your thyroid health and hormone balance.[35] Start small and keep it simple: Swap a few toxic household and personal care products for natural alternatives each week, using the list of main thyroid offenders (see page 190 to help focus your efforts.

LET'S BREAK IT DOWN

- Estrogen dominance and the symptoms of low thyroid function are common hormonal imbalances in women of all ages due both to lifestyle and environmental factors. Encouraging hormone balance will help you get the results from intermittent fasting that you're looking for.

- Estrogen is required for optimal function of almost every organ in your body—from your brain to your bladder, bones, and heart—which is why an imbalance leads to wide-ranging symptoms, from weight gain and bloating to period problems and mood swings.

- Thyroid-related conditions are widespread among women and are too often underrecognized and underdiagnosed. Supporting the thyroid and the healthy functioning of thyroid hormones and reducing overall inflammation are essential wellness practices.

- Reducing your exposure to endocrine-disrupting chemicals as much as possible is one of the most powerful ways you can support estrogen and thyroid hormone balance.

Part 4

MAKE IT A LIFESTYLE

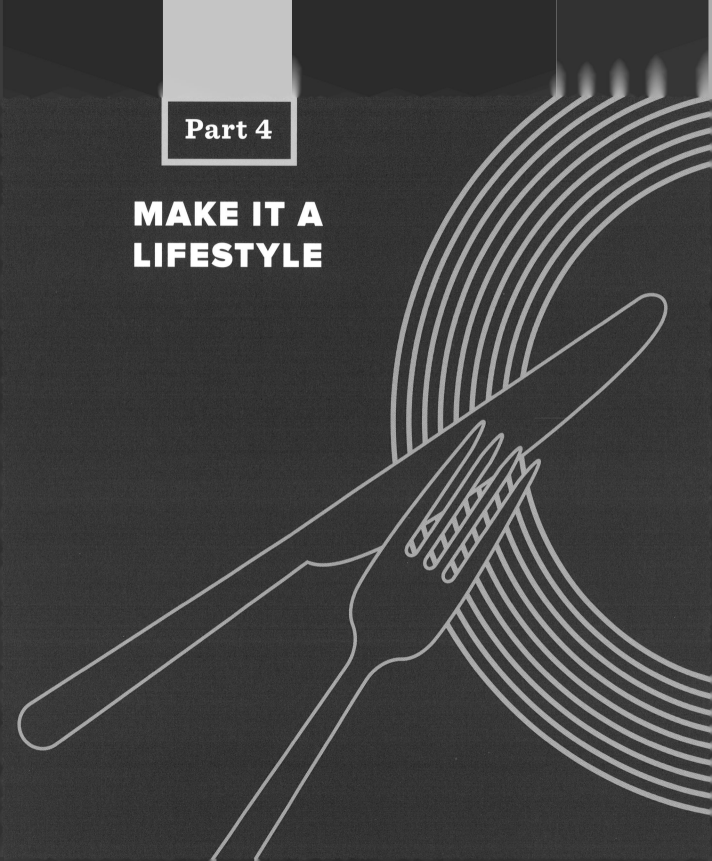

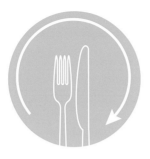

CHAPTER 12

Maintain Motivation

When you go through any kind of transformation, you will experience ups and downs and unexpected challenges. Just when you think you've got it all figured out, suddenly you're lost. It's okay. It happens. I'll share strategies to help you maintain motivation no matter what comes your way, as well as ways to stay focused on your health and wellness goals without losing sight of everything else in your life that matters, too.

Losing more than 100 pounds (45.3 kg) was more than a radical physical transformation for me; it was also a mental transformation. The mental and physical aspects go hand in hand and, in a lot of ways, the physical transformation may have stayed out of reach if I hadn't addressed my mind-set. How we approach stress is a determining factor in how successful we'll be at sticking with any endeavor, including intermittent fasting, over the long term. I probably don't have to tell you that stress is the number-one threat to motivation. It will sap and stall you. It can ruin you, making it easier for you to make bad decisions and poor choices that don't align with what you really want. We can't escape stress, but we can change our perception of it.

Beat Burnout

How did I get to be over 300 pounds (136 kg)? Burnout. I was stressed out and so focused on my career and making money to take care of my family that I lost sight of the big picture, or what I call "The Four Pillars":

1. Health

2. Family

3. Career

4. Spirituality

Once you stop attending to a pillar, it starts to crumble and then weakens all the other pillars. Pretty soon, they all come crashing down, and that's right about where I was when I topped out at my heaviest—depressed and miserable.

Where I went wrong was trying to find balance. Balance is a joke. You can't find balance. Why? You cannot be everything at once. You cannot be a superstar parent, top CEO, jacked athlete, and devout individual all at the same time. And, when you try, you end up with four weak pillars. Balance means putting 25 percent into each pillar. That's not good enough—for your own sense of meaning, satisfaction, or accomplishment, or for the people you love.

I chased my career and success in business and also tried to be a super husband because I was filled with the fear I would lose my family while pursuing success. Problem was, I ended up being a cruddy executive and a cruddy partner. With my career and family pillars wobbling, I was stressed—and started eating. Pretty soon, I'd gained 100 pounds (45.3 kg). I took a jackhammer to my health pillar. And my spirituality? Out the window. It wasn't long before my whole life came crashing down.

Striving for balance was fighting to become someone I could never possibly be and burning me out in the process. Our brains don't have the ability to multitask or do more than one task with sufficient focus.[1] It's impossible for me to focus on being an amazing husband

and father at the same time that I'm focusing on running my business, what I should eat, and my spirituality. My brain just can't do it all at once. What the brain can do is task switch, shifting between activities.

Here's what I should have done: Give 100 percent to one pillar at any given moment. Now, when I'm at work, I'm 100 percent at work. Each nanosecond, my focus is on the task at hand. But, if my wife calls, my focus shifts to her. While we're speaking, I'm 100 percent focused on the family pillar. During my workout, I tune in to my body 100 percent. Those moments I spend in reflection or meditation absorb 100 percent of my awareness. Second by second, I am all in on one pillar. My mind does not deviate. I redirect my attention as needed, for sure, but always with one target in my sight, not several. There is nothing else on my mind other than what is right in front of me that very second.

Don't get me wrong—it's difficult. We're all flooded by information and demands on our attention constantly. But, by living in the moment, you'll find that your health will improve, your family will be happier, your business will prosper, and you'll be more in touch with your spirituality.

The key to maintaining all Four Pillars is scheduling time for each one, and that doesn't mean you have to block out space for all four every day (though that would be great). It does mean looking at your daily, weekly, or monthly calendar and making sure you have health, family, career, and spirituality time represented. Ask yourself, "When will my family

TOP TACTIC

LIVE IN THE MOMENT

Try it: For the next two days, focus on thinking only about what is happening at that very second. When you hug a loved one, be 100 percent present. Don't let thoughts of work cloud that moment. When you open the refrigerator to make dinner, have nothing else on your mind but the foods you want to choose. Notice when your mind drifts. What do those moments tell you? What can you do to bring your attention back to the present moment?

time be?" And, so on, until you have hours committed to all the pillars.

Without a plan, I guarantee that a pillar will be overlooked, and probably more than one. Flying by the seat of your pants every day is a recipe for even more severe burnout than searching for that elusive balance. Instead, use your calendar and dive, 100 percent, into supporting the goals and people you care about, while being sincerely effective at doing so.

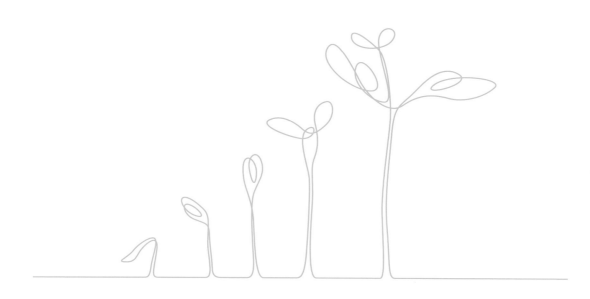

Adopt a Growth Mind-Set

We know now that the human brain is capable of growing new brain cells and forming new neural connections. If the brain is functioning properly, it is constantly evolving and changing, enabling us to learn, improve existing capabilities, and develop new skills all the time. Simply put, your brain—you—always has room to grow. Adopting a growth mind-set means acknowledging this fact and allowing it to shape your perspective.

It's too easy to get stuck in a fixed mind-set, thinking nothing is ever going to change. Maybe you've been trying to extend your fast but just can't seem to make it that additional hour. If you have a fixed mind-set, you think: *I'll never be able to do this. I'm just a failure and that's how it's always going to be. I might as well just give up on this whole intermittent fasting thing right now.* A fixed mind-set keeps you small.

With a growth mind-set, you think: *What can I learn from this? How can I use what my body is telling me to develop a new strategy? Maybe extending my fast isn't the way to go right now and, instead, I should try adding a HIIT workout to my current fasting length and see how that influences my results.* A growth mind-set encourages you to evolve.

We all face setbacks, plateaus, and disappointments. There's no way to sugarcoat that. However, we can make a conscious choice to approach difficult situations with a growth mind-set and use those challenges to get closer to who we wish to be.

When it's time to open that pantry door and grab something to eat, yes, you should be 100 percent in the game. But, while you're filling out an expense report or helping your kids with schoolwork, you should not be thinking about the turkey sticks you (maybe) ate one too many of two hours earlier. If you notice you are 100 percent focused on your health, especially your diet, 100 percent of the time, consider seeking help from a health care provider or trained therapist. Orthorexia is an unhealthy obsession with healthy eating and should not be ignored.

The people you spend the most time with are a major influence on who you are. Surround yourself with individuals who support your health and wellness goals. They'll keep you motivated, accountable, and upbeat. You may already have that community. If your current friends and family are on board and eager to support you enthusiastically, or even join your efforts, congratulations—but don't hesitate to look beyond your existing circle.

Branch Out

Now is always a good time to branch out and make new friends who live in alignment with your lifestyle. No matter where you are on your transformation journey, it helps to know people in the same circumstances. Dipping a toe into intermittent fasting? Check. Experimenting with extended fasting? Check. Not sure of the best way to work out? Check. No matter the type of support or advice you're looking for, you can find it either online or IRL. As I started spending more time at the gym and health food store, I started meeting new people and, almost before I knew it, I had a new circle. Don't miss out on the benefits of community.

Choose Supportive Relationships

Part of creating a new community involves reevaluating current relationships. Now that you're making changes to your lifestyle, you may notice that certain friends, family members, or colleagues who you regularly spend time with are no longer the best fit for you and the attitudes you want to be around. I hate to break it to you but, in my experience, the majority of them aren't going to be accepting of your new lifestyle, and whatever their reasons, don't dwell in relationships that no longer serve you or allow their negative mindset to rub off on you. Easier said than done, I know. But, distancing yourself from toxic people and creating boundaries (or breaking things off completely) may be the only way to restore your health and well-being.

Be Okay with Being Alone

Early in my health journey, I didn't want to be alone, so I continued to surround myself with people I thought would comfort me—but all they did was bring me down because they weren't on the same mission I was on. I should have accepted the fact that it's okay to be alone and that you can be alone without being lonely. Sometimes, you're the best company you'll ever have.

TOP TACTIC

LEARN TO LOVE THE ANGER DRIVE

Anger, controlled and in bursts, can propel you toward your goals. We're talking about strategic anger here, not out-of-your-mind or self-destructive rages. You cannot live on anger, but you can use it to your advantage.

See, when I gained weight, I also gained stretch marks. Now that I've lost weight, you can see them all over my body. They make me angry, furious really, that I was so negligent with my health and allowed my life to become so out of control. Instead of wallowing in that anger and letting it distract me, I use it as a quick pick-me-up to stay focused on all the positives that have come out of those stretch marks and all the good things I hope to accomplish in the future. Don't be afraid of your anger; you have to be real with your emotions. Use it as a shot in the arm to get you through the challenges.

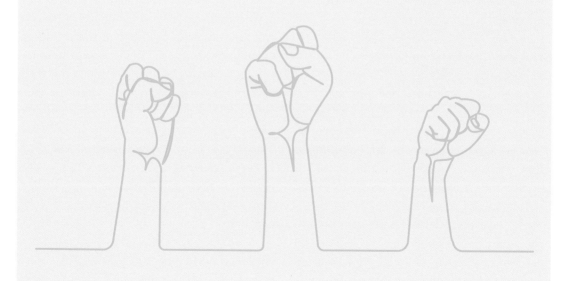

One main reason motivation lags is because we've hit some sort of roadblock, such as a weight loss plateau, or boredom has struck and we're just not that into intermittent fasting or working out. What to do? Use this five-step strategy to bust through those roadblocks, spark true motivation, and reinvigorate your intermittent fasting lifestyle.

Step One: Register Reality

Be real with yourself and what's going on. You've gotten off track. You're frustrated that you're not losing weight. You feel guilty for missing your workouts last week. Own what's happening and own your emotions. Look, the struggle is real, but being in denial puts a wall between you and reality and makes it impossible to address what's going on and strategize solutions.

Step Two: Set Micro Goals

Our bodies and brains are goal oriented. Simply by setting small goals for yourself, you can harness the power of your body's natural reward system. When we expect to receive a reward, the brain releases the neurotransmitter dopamine, heightening our sense of pleasure and reinforcing our desire to experience that bliss again.[2]

Let's say your goal is to get back into a gym routine. Set a clearly defined, achievable goal: Get to the gym at 7 a.m. Next, write it down. Yes, that helps make it more tangible, but it also crystallizes the goal in your mind, so that when you successfully walk through that gym door at 7:00 a.m., your brain triggers the reward system, and you get a surge of dopamine. That sense of reward and pleasure makes you want to meet that goal again—and again. Your body takes it from there, producing more dopamine, providing a steady influx of motivation.

Step Three: Use Visualization

Visualization, creating a mental image of a future desired outcome, is an exceptionally effective way to maintain motivation and achieve your goals. Visualization is not about magical thinking or faking it until you make it. Visualization works because it creates new neural pathways in your brain that set you up to do what you've imagined doing.[3]

The neurons in your brain can't tell the difference between an actual event and an event you visualized. They interpret a mental image, for example of you entering the gym, the same as a real-life action. When you visualize walking into the facility, your neurons create a pathway to perform the action, even though your body doesn't move a muscle. It's like your brain has done a dress rehearsal and now your body is primed and ready to perform the physical motions involved in arriving at the gym.

Visualization has long been associated with improved performance. Research has shown that training by mentally moving parts of the body is almost as effective as true physical movement.[4] Putting our minds to something makes it easier for us to achieve it.

With visualization, though, it's not good enough to just picture a moment in your mind; you need to truly believe it. You want to use all your senses and create as much detail as possible to create a strong emotional connection to the outcome. There are two types of visualizations:

Outcome visualization is the process of seeing yourself accomplishing your goal—what it looks like, smells like, tastes like, sounds like, and feels like.

Process visualization is seeing yourself completing each step necessary to achieve your desired outcome. If your goal is to start intermittent fasting again after a break, visualize preparing your pre-fast meal, drinking your apple cider vinegar lemonade in the morning, doing your workout, dealing with mid-fast hunger, and breaking the fast.

Use both types of visualization to create a vivid mental image to motivate and energize you and build your confidence so you can believe these results are attainable and get your brain ready to make it happen.

Step Four: Take Action

Take one action. If you've been using visualization, you've already marked a trail that will make acting easier. But you still have to walk the walk.

Piggyback on visualization by using visual cues to spur you on. A visual cue, such as setting your gym bag by the front door, is registered by a part of the brain called the rhinal cortex, which translates the image into a signal for action.[5] That bag is not just a reminder; it's actually going to get you in the mood for showing up and working out.

There's no "right" or perfect time to start. Take *this* moment to take one clear action that will move you closer to your goal. That one action has the power to start a positive chain of events, leading to more positive changes, thanks to your body's innate reward system. For example, add a few circuits of strength training to your workout routine while fasting, or add a long walk during your fasting window. You'll feel so good that you'll be more likely to pay extra attention to breaking your fast properly. The more energized you feel from fasting, the more you'll want to get back into an intermittent fasting lifestyle and find ways to maximize your workouts to keep the physical and emotional benefits coming.

Step Five: Recognize Success

Time to get real again. Take stock. Are things moving in the right direction? Monitor your progress regularly. Research has shown that the more often you monitor your progress, the greater the likelihood you will succeed.[6] You'll be more attuned to where you need a new strategy or extra support as well as what's working well. Above all, be sure to celebrate the small wins, no matter how small they seem. Those small victories have been shown to boost motivation and self-confidence just as much as the big ones.[7]

One way to reignite your motivation to go to the gym is to start working out at the same time every day.[8] Researchers found that a strong instigation habit, or cue that reliably prompts exercise, successfully predicted long-term consistency in workouts. The end, or start, of your work day may be just the signaling you need, or try an alarm clock or a visual cue. By creating a habit, you'll go for your run or do your strength training without even thinking about it. Don't get stuck in the rut of doing the same routine every day, though—this same study found no benefit to repeating the same exercises over time.

TOP TACTIC

TAKE A BREAK

You've hit a weight-loss plateau. You've tried all sorts of ways to supercharge your results, such as mixing things up (see chapter 8), but nothing has worked. Try a two-week fasting break. Eat your normal amount of calories but give fasting a rest. One study compared participants who consistently cut their calories by one-third for sixteen straight weeks to those participants who followed the same reduced-calorie diet, but for two weeks on and two weeks off, for a total of sixteen weeks of dieting. The group that took breaks ended up losing significantly more weight and fat. The intermittent dieters had an average weight loss of 31 pounds (14 kg) and fat mass loss of 27.1 pounds (12.29 kg), whereas the consistent dieters lost 20 pounds (9 kg) with an average fat mass loss of 9.2 pounds (4.17 kg). The intermittent dieters also experienced an increase in their resting energy expenditure, or how much energy the body burns at rest, spreading the potential weight loss gap even further.[9] Taking a little break now and then is powerful and can make the difference you're looking for.

ACKNOWLEDGE IT'S OKAY

It is okay to be real with your emotions. It's okay to look in the mirror and dislike what you see. That anger drive will push you forward.

It's okay to be angry with others. It happens. You're going to snap at your partner. You're going to deflect and blame them for breaking your fast earlier than you planned, or for not having your fast-breaking foods in the fridge, or whatever. Acknowledge what you're feeling, apologize for lashing out, and commit to feeling but not acting out on your anger again.

It's okay to have mood swings. Our bodies are always changing. We will have ups and downs. Period.

It's all okay as long as you own your emotions and believe, deep down, that there's nothing you can't handle.

LET'S BREAK IT DOWN

- How we approach stress is a determining factor in how successful we'll be at sticking with any endeavor, including intermittent fasting, over the long term.

- Beat burnout by living in the moment, dedicating 100 percent of your focus to one of The Four Pillars (health, family, career, spirituality) in any given nanosecond.

- Face setbacks, plateaus, and disappointments with a growth mind-set and use these challenges to get closer to who you wish to be.

- Find a supportive community of people who live in alignment with your health goals and values.

- Use my five-step strategy to spark true motivation and reinvigorate your intermittent fasting lifestyle no matter the roadblock in your path.

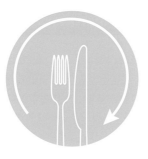

CHAPTER 13

Include Your Family

The best way to make intermittent fasting a lifestyle is to get your family, the people who share your home and daily life, on board with it. This doesn't mean your significant other or other adult family members need to fast, too—though, once they notice how much better you look and feel, they may want to jump in. But there are ways you can actively create the kind of supportive, loving home environment that will help sustain your healthy lifestyle changes while strengthening your relationships with family members. And, although children and adolescents should *not* do intermittent fasting, they can certainly reap the benefits of all you know about eating clean and having you as a positive role model.

Communication is the key to avoiding relationship stress, especially with your partner or other adults closest to you. You don't need to shout from the rooftops that you're intermittent fasting, but your new eating style won't go unnoticed by those in your home. Don't lie or keep them in the dark. Being secretive breeds worry and discomfort. You want others to be informed and on your side.

Explain the Changes You Are Making and Share Your Plans and Goals

Be clear and kind: *I'm committed to trying intermittent fasting and eating more whole foods as part of living a healthier lifestyle. I'm going to start fasting for sixteen hours, three times a week, which means I'll be skipping breakfast on those mornings, but I'd still like to have coffee together. After a month, I'm going to assess my weight and body composition to determine how well intermittent fasting works for me.*

Share the Reasons You Are Making These Changes

Maybe you had a health scare or don't like what you see in the mirror. Maybe you've decided to try intermittent fasting so you can be a better overall version of you. Don't hesitate to let your family know the reason for your decisions. My family certainly is the reason for me. I want to be the best husband and father I can be and run around with my kids and wife

for as long as possible. Being overweight and unhealthy puts that goal at risk. My family is a major motivation for maintaining my intermittent fasting lifestyle and, by sharing that with them, they know everything I'm doing is for not only for me but for them, too.

Be Candid About What May Change and What Will Stay the Same

Change can be difficult, especially when one person in a family is changing and the others aren't. A frequent major pain point for significant others centers on how much of your time they think these changes will consume, potentially putting added responsibilities on them or taking away from family time together. Try to troubleshoot this in advance. For example: You're planning to skip dinner a few nights each week, but you're the household chef. Reassure your family that you're comfortable preparing the meal, even though you won't be eating it, or you will prep it the night before so it's ready for your partner to heat and serve, or another solution to help ease the transition and find reasonable compromises for everyone. Be respectful of your family members' time and do your best to find mutually agreeable solutions.

Ask for Support

Be honest and upfront about how your family can be there for you. On the emotional side that could mean: *I'm making these changes to improve my health and I'd really appreciate your love, understanding, and support.* On the more practical side: *Could you get the kids ready in the morning one day each week while I go for a run?* Or, *It's tough for me to do the food shopping during my fasting window. Could you do the food shopping, or arrange for the groceries to be delivered, one day each week to help me out?*

Prepare for Questions

Answer questions calmly. Don't get defensive. If your loved ones ask questions, it's because they care. Getting comfortable with the science of intermittent fasting, how it works, and its benefits is a huge help when faced with questions such as, "Won't your metabolism slow down?" or, "Isn't skipping meals dangerous?" (Refer to chapters 1 through 3.) If you don't know the answer, tell them you'll find the information requested and share what you learn. There are many online resources written by respected experts, including my videos, to turn to. (Start with the videos available at FastingIsEasy.com.) The point isn't to bombard your family and loved ones with information or try to convince them of the merits of intermittent fasting, but, rather, to keep them updated on what you're doing, why you're doing it, and respectfully, responsibly answer their questions. They may have concerns or raise points you hadn't thought of. With a growth mind-set, you can use their feedback as a way to learn more.

When it comes to questions from kids, keep it age appropriate. All they may need to hear is that your adult body has different needs than their growing one.

With science on your side, you can be confident about intermittent fasting. Your loved ones want what's best for you. Make it easy for them to see why intermittent fasting is.

Listen to Concerns

I'm worried you'll be too lightheaded/ grouchy/tired/hungry to go to work/coach the kids' soccer team/volunteer at the food pantry. Take others' concerns seriously and reassure your family that your intention with intermittent fasting is to become an even better, more involved member of the family.

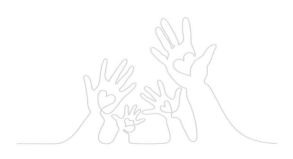

The most important thing you can do while making a lifestyle change is to love your family more. You want your family associating these changes with a person who is more loving, more present, more attentive, more respectful, and more grateful for having them. Experiencing what a positive influence these changes are will make your family more likely to embrace your new lifestyle and want to be part of it. Think about it: If you turn into a total jerk and disconnect from family life, how likely is it that your family will support intermittent fasting? Yeah, not very.

Share Mealtimes

Even if a meal falls during your fasting window, be present. You can bond with your family without breaking your fast. You don't have to remove yourself from the family dynamic or eat when everyone else eats. Don't miss out on this valuable bonding and togetherness time. Sit down. Enjoy a fasting-friendly beverage and participate in the conversation and time together. At first, you might find it challenging to sip on green tea or sparkling water while your family digs in, but you'll soon appreciate that it's the laughing, chatting, and engaging that makes this time special, not the eating.

Attend Family Events, Holidays, and Special Occasions

Celebrations are what make life worth living. I urge you not to skip them. You may decide to go off schedule and forego your usual fast if it falls over a wedding, vacation, or birthday bash. Or you may decide fasting is the best thing for you and you'll negotiate the event in a fasted state. You're in control. It's up to you. One of the best things about intermittent fasting is the flexibility it gives you. When and how you fast is entirely up to you.

If you're fasting, rest assured you can still be social, catching up, sharing news, giving gifts, dancing, playing games, and making memories. There are lots of ways to bond without eating. A simple ready response like, "I'm not hungry right now, maybe later. I'll just have some sparkling water," is usually enough to shut down even the most persistent food pusher.

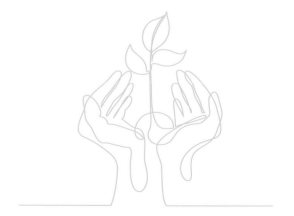

TOP TACTIC

EMPOWER YOUR KIDS

Show kids how to:

- ✓ **Make their own breakfast.** This can help you get up and go without inadvertently breaking your fast in the morning while also building your child's sense of accomplishment and self-confidence.

- ✓ **Read a food label.** It's never too soon to start recognizing certifications such as USDA organic or learning about ingredients and nutritional content to use to compare options. Share how you make choices so kids can learn to do the same for themselves.

COME TOGETHER

Make it easy for your family to spend time with you. You don't have to go on this new health journey alone and you really, really shouldn't.

Invite (Don't Nag)

People do not respond well to nagging or being made to feel as though they are somehow, suddenly, on the wrong side with their food and lifestyle choices. Your family doesn't need to change their ways, but give them the opportunity to find out more about what you're doing and participate, if desired. That could mean leaving the door open for them to do a fast, make a meal, or work out with you. They may not take you up on any of your offers at first—or ever—but leave the door open. Respect your family members' right to choose what's best for their bodies without discounting or devaluing where they are on their journey while carrying on with what you know is best for yours.

Share Foods That Are Good for You and the Whole Family

Food doesn't have to be a you-vs.-them stand-off. And, although you may want to clear out the fridge and cupboards to make way for all of your fasting-friendly foods, don't try to turn your whole household's eating style on its head at once. Try adding, not subtracting. Eating clean is good for everyone. Having an abundance of lean protein and fresh whole foods readily available will help you break your fast properly and offer your family nutritious meal choices. Offer new foods for everyone to try: Green tea, turkey jerky, and top-notch coffee anyone?

Be Active Together

We could all stand to move more. Your new habit of going to the gym or working out regularly may motivate your partner to be more physically active, too. Invite them along to your sessions and encourage them to find activities that make them feel good. You don't have to do the same workout to get the benefits of working out together. You don't even have to do a workout. Get the whole family energized with everything from a living room dance party or game of tag to a walk around the neighborhood, hike in a local park (bring the dog!), yoga stretches, or swim time. Make it fun—for you and them.

BE POSITIVE

You feel good, right? Just living your life in the way that's best for you and that promotes your health, energy, and optimism sends a powerful and positive message. You're leading by example, modeling behavior that you hope rubs off on your loved ones, such as being physically active and eating fresh whole, nutrient-dense foods with intention and awareness. I live a healthy lifestyle to set an example for my children so they don't become a statistic. I want them to see and experience the world as I do now, not through that miserable, discontented lens through which I viewed the world ten years ago at 300 pounds (136 kg). Being the best version of yourself will indirectly affect everyone around you.

LET'S BREAK IT DOWN

- The best way to make intermittent fasting a lifestyle is to get your family, the people who share your home and daily life, on board for support.

- Keep the lines of communication open. Be clear and kind about the changes you are making and why. Answer questions about your new lifestyle calmly and with science-backed support. Listen to concerns and work with your family to address them responsibly.

- Love your family more so they associate your new lifestyle with a person who is the very best version of you: more present, more attentive, more grateful.

- Invite your family to come on this journey with you but don't nag or expect them to follow your lead. Respect them and their decisions while taking care of yourself.

- Lead by example.

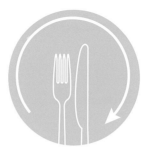

CHAPTER 14

Do What's Best for You

Look. There are a lot of voices out there telling you what's best for you. You should know that modern diet and fitness culture is hyperfocused on how you should look, not your health or feeling good inside. And everything your doctor tells you isn't always the best advice for you. This means you need to be your own advocate, and that starts with listening to your body and honoring your goals, which, of course, may shift over time as you get older or your life circumstances change. That's fine. You can adapt and adjust intermittent fasting to work for you over the long term. Just be prepared for the haters. Ignore them. Do it for you and nobody else. Do what makes you feel good. Do what's best for you.

LISTEN TO YOUR BODY AND HONOR YOUR GOALS

There's no one way to approach a healthy lifestyle—only the way that's right for you. This applies to intermittent fasting, eating styles, workouts, supplements, and so on. Living a healthy lifestyle means gaining the confidence to know what's right for you and choosing to follow that path.

Nobody Knows You Like You Do

Only you know what feels good to you, mentally and physically. Only you can hear the messages your body sends to let you know what's working right, what isn't, and what needs immediate attention. Not your mother. Not your partner. Not your boss. Not a health guru. Not a doctor. No one. You are the expert on you.

Be Your Own Advocate

There is a flood of diet and nutrition advice coming at us all the time. I'm overwhelmed by it, too! New studies and strategies hit the headlines daily. Talking heads promote the latest trends nonstop all over social media. On the flipside, it can seem as if the medical community is behind the times, stuck in old thinking about calories in/calories out being the be-all and end-all of weight loss and woefully out of date because of the limited nutrition education most doctors receive in medical school.[1]

Be your own advocate. Start making the changes you've been wanting to make now. Don't wait for someone else to tell you it's time. Practice due diligence—checking sources, claims, and studies. Learn as much as you can from legitimate, respected sources to support your efforts. Own your body and your health by owning your education. All the noise in the health space can drown out the excellent, insightful research being done. Find the outlets you trust and don't blindly follow anyone's recommendation.

Keep It Real

Real health is feeling good, energized, upbeat. Sure, looking fit and attractive on the outside is nice, too, but external appearance should not be the only focus of living a healthy lifestyle. The difficulty with keeping it real is that the majority of the diet and fitness industry emphasizes what's on the outside without paying enough attention to what's on the inside. We're held to standards that are entirely impossible to uphold and, most of the time, the jacked bodies we're shown aren't even real. They're air-brushed, hair-and-makeup phonies, probably on performance enhancements.

I've done some work in the fitness industry. At one time, I made it my mission to get on a fitness magazine cover and, ultimately, appeared on five. I quickly realized that staying in that world any longer wasn't for me. It was too shallow and narcissistic and filled with people overcompensating for their insecurities but never really focusing on health or truly feeling good. It started to turn me into a monster and away from the original reasons I started working out in the first place.

There's a lot of propaganda out there that will lead you to believe a six-pack is what matters most. Don't opt in. We do not have to live up to whatever ideal the industry is selling at the moment. Fitness is not necessarily health. Keep it real. Being healthy is always in style.

You Don't Have to Be Strict 100 Percent of the Time

You do want to be strict during your fasting window to get the benefits of the fast, but you don't need to be inflexible with your intermittent fasting schedule or always eat clean or never snack. There are two reasons for this:

1. You're human—and humans are not perfect. Holding yourself to the standard of perfection will lead to failure and resentment. There have been times when I've been so strict and buttoned up I couldn't live a normal life. My pillars began to crumble. I'd pushed myself so far in one direction that, like a rubber band, I snapped right back the other way. Give yourself some space.

2. Intermittent fasting works because spontaneous calorie restriction shocks the body. Boom! It's not about progressive calorie restriction. So, you don't want to consistently limit calories or always be on a fast. Having a "cheat" meal once in a while isn't going to ruin you. You want a contrast between high and low calories.

WAYS TO DEAL WITH NEGATIVE COMMENTS ON SOCIAL MEDIA

Keep calm and think through your next steps before acting and know what you hope to achieve. Sometimes a response is called for; other times, staying silent is the best way to defang negativity.

- Block and delete, if you are being bullied, harassed, or threatened, or if you've had enough of being insulted.

- Ignore trolls, comments with no substance behind them, or comments you can let roll off your back.

- Respond, if you feel you need to set the record straight or protect your reputation. Be positive and polite and stick to facts you can support. Don't be baited into an extended back-and-forth argument with someone who doesn't really want to hear your thoughts anyway.

One of the worst pieces of advice I heard when I was going through my transformation was, "Don't lose weight too fast." At first glance that sounds like a reasonable, responsible recommendation, right? We've all watched someone lose a ton of weight quickly only to have it pile back on even faster. There is nothing wrong with slow and steady, but it's not your only option. You can lose fat more efficiently without losing muscle or tanking your metabolism, which we know will set you up for rebounding weight gain, with intermittent fasting than with other protocols. The keto diet is another good option. In one study, participants who lost 45 pounds (20 kg) in four months on a ketogenic diet showed no change in the resting metabolic rate.[2] You have options.

Lose weight at the pace *you* want.

ADAPT AS NEEDED

Your health journey is just that, a journey. A process. There's no fixed way forward or end point. Change is going to happen. Roll with it.

Goals change. Mine certainly have. At one point, I was very into building muscle. Now, that's not my priority. I want to be able to roll around on the ground with my son and my daughter and play in the park with my family and not end up with an aching back because I'm carrying a bunch of muscle. I'm about 10 pounds (4.5 kg) lighter than I once was and my face appears thinner. Is one way of being better than the other? No. One just suits my current lifestyle and goals better, and I've revised my eating and workout routine to reflect the body I want now.

My goals and lifestyle will inevitably change again. Yours will, too, and the key is to adjust along with the changes. I'll adapt to be healthy while staying in alignment with what's happening in my life in that moment. I do what works for me at a given point in time knowing it may not always work for me. Intermittent fasting remains a consistent part of my healthy lifestyle because of how adaptable it is. Different fasting window lengths suit a variety of goals and schedules. (Also subject to change!) Even though some things change, intermittent fasting can be a constant on your journey.

As goals change so, too, will your body change. We can't stop time no matter what the beauty bloggers say, and with the passage of time comes changes. You may need extra support to maintain lean muscle mass and bone density. Hormone levels shift.[3] The composition of your gut microbiome may alter.[4] Pregnancy, illness, a chronic health condition, or an injury can affect your body in a multitude of subtle and not-so-subtle ways. By acknowledging these changes, we can modify our approaches to healthy living to suit our new needs. La-La Land does us no good here, either. You may need to fast for shorter periods, take a break, or revamp your diet. Work with your body, not against it.

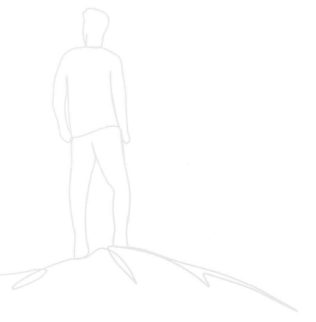

IGNORE THE HATERS

Get ready. They're everywhere, especially on social media. Their animosity can either compel you to continue doing what you're doing with fortitude and strength or push you to throw in the towel. Don't let what's going on with them undermine you. Overcoming negativity and judgment is exhausting, but it's a lot easier if you're prepared.

People Will Judge You

They'll judge you for being too fat, too skinny, too muscular, or not muscular enough. For losing weight. For losing weight and then gaining some of it back. For being or doing what they consider "unhealthy" and for being or doing what you know to be "healthy." For not looking beautiful and shiny enough. We're not talking about genuine concern here—people asking you how you're doing and listening to what you tell them with compassion. No, we're talking about people who simply want to spit hate and hurl negative comments to hurt you or take you down a peg.

> *"I'd lose weight, too, if I were starving myself!"*

> *"Oh, I thought you were intermittent fasting. Why are you drinking coffee or sprinkling cinnamon in your water?"*

> *"You're not fasting; you're not doing it correctly."*

> *"You'll never keep the weight off."*

Or they forget you're a human being who gets sick, has dark circles after a rough night of sleep, or can look a little bloated. Getting ill or looking less than your best doesn't mean you're a failure or prove that intermittent fasting is terrible for you or that you're unhealthy. It just means you're human like everyone else. But haters don't see it that way. They're looking for ways to take you down, and believe me, they'll find them.

Then, there are the people who just think you're weird. A strange, perplexing outlier who is too different to be around, or who pushes their buttons in the wrong way.

Who knows what provokes folks to air this abuse? Could be jealousy or insecurity. They know losing weight or improving your fitness takes hard work, but they want to minimize that work by saying you had help or took supplements or "cheated" in this or that way.

It doesn't really matter why—their motivations are not worth a second of your time. What does matter is what you do with those comments. No matter how thick your skin, hate hurts. It can stress you out, making you second-guess yourself and lose confidence in your choices. Don't let that happen. Ignore them if you can or recognize how malicious and painful they are and put them aside. You are not their comments. You are not what they think of you. You are the expert on you, and you know what's best for you. Period.

Some of the best advice I've been given is: Drive yourself; don't be driven. Don't let others direct your life. You're in the driver's seat.

Let people think you're weird or whatever they want all while you get in the best shape of your life.

Enjoy What You Do

Take pleasure in intermittent fasting and clean eating—not just the results, but the experience, too. I love learning about what's happening inside my body at the cellular level. I'm excited by new findings in nutrition science. Hopefully, after reading this book, you've become more interested in these things, too. The point is, I don't just tolerate or put up with my lifestyle—I get a kick out of it. Not every moment of a fast is bliss but, big picture, everything I'm doing to stay healthy is something I enjoy doing and learning about. Find the joy in your approach and invest in strategies that you genuinely care about. Enjoying what you do will get you through the rough times and the naysayers.

Be Inspired by Your Story

We all have scars, visible reminders of our story and signs of change. We may feel the need to hide them, but I propose that you be inspired by them instead. To see your scars in the way I see my stretch marks, as encouragement to keep to your path. I'm proud of my stretch marks. They indicate survival, and I appreciate what I've accomplished to get them: a healthier body, a growing business, and a top YouTube channel that helps millions of people. It's my opinion of those stretch marks that matters, and I choose to let those scars keep me motivated. Whenever I take a hot shower and the water turns my skin red, but my stretch marks remain pale white, I can see plainly why I do what I do.

No matter what your scar is, let it inspire you and manifest a true, driving power inside you that you can use to accomplish the goals you set for yourself. Let it remind you that yours is the only opinion that matters.

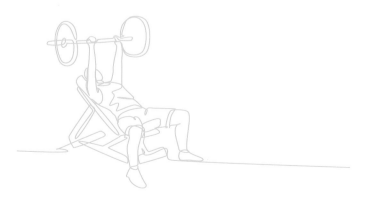

LET'S BREAK IT DOWN

- There are a lot of voices telling you what's best for you, but your voice is the one that matters. You are the expert on you and what's best for you.

- Keep it real by focusing on true health and feeling good, not external appearances.

- Allow yourself to be human and don't hold yourself to an impossible standard of perfection.

- Recognize that your goals *and* your body will change—it's inevitable—and you have tools, such as intermittent fasting, to help you adapt.

- Ignore the haters and find inspiration and motivation in your story.

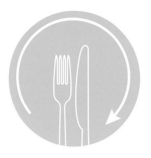

CONCLUSION

I'm Here for You

I'm passionate about intermittent fasting because I know it works, and it is one of the most effective ways to remake your body composition, revitalize your health, and upgrade your life. And, although we've covered a lot of ground and nuance over the course of this book, the fundamentals are straightforward. When in doubt, keep it simple and add refinements as you grow more comfortable.

Don't get discouraged if you hit a few bumps in the road. Return to this book for encouragement and real-world advice to help smooth your path. I hope you'll also tune in to my YouTube channel for more of the same, plus additional information about how to fast effectively and efficiently and eat to support your goals based on the remarkable research that continues to excite me each and every

day. All the time, I'm learning new things that help me take care of my body better. And my mission remains the same: to share what I learn with you. The more you know about your body and what works (and doesn't work) for you, the more fun you'll have living a healthy lifestyle, and the easier it will be.

Nothing is more satisfying to me than hearing from people who have transformed their bodies and lives because of the studies and advice I've shared. If you see me in a coffee shop or at the airport, don't hesitate to come on up to me and say hello. Making a positive impact with what I know, and connecting with others striving to reach their full potential, is why I do what I do. You, too, can have a positive influence on those around you, especially your children. The more we show our kids how amazing their bodies are and what they can do when they care for them properly, the better off we'll all be. At the end of the day, if you perform better, the world performs better. I'm so happy that you're now part of this pioneering intermittent fasting and nutrition community.

Becoming the best version of you starts with the decisions you make each day, right now. You can't undo choices you made in the past or predict where you'll be in the future. But, in this very second, you have the power to make choices that can define who you are and who you'll become. No matter where you are on your journey, take this moment to choose your health.

I will be here for you.

Acknowledgments

To my children, who have taught me more than I ever could have imagined about life. For reminding me that life is much more than what meets the eye and for giving me a purpose other than myself.

To my thoughtful and mesmerizing wife, Amber, who has never judged me, even in my worst of times, but has only provided me a place to think safely and securely to work through my struggles—all while offering a shoulder to cry on.

To my father, whom I didn't become close to until later in life, when it was almost too late. For showing me how to be a father, long after he passed away. I have learned more from you after your passing than I ever could have imagined, and you've made me a better dad.

To the mountains, for always being my safe place and where I go in my mind when the going gets tough.

To the ocean, for always being tumultuous even when you're seemingly calm. You're inspiring and intimidating, yet healing and breaking.

To Timmy, Remi, Kolt, and Bo, our four pups, who have always shown us how to share compassion in a way that some find invisible. You've always been by my side through the craziest adventures.

To the open road, thank you for giving me the opportunity to think, to heal, to talk. The most life-changing discussions have happened with the double yellow in front of me. There is no way I would be where I am today without the open road.

About the Author

THOMAS DELAUER is a celebrity fitness and nutrition expert and social media influencer. Early in his career, as a busy executive in the health care space, Thomas tipped the scales at almost 300 pounds (136 kg). He was prediabetic, hypertensive, and battling severe depression and anxiety. With the encouragement and guidance of some of the physicians he worked with and managed, Thomas lost more than 100 pounds (45.3 kg) and regained his health with intermittent fasting, the ketogenic diet, and exercise in a little over one year.

Excited by everything he'd learned and determined not to go back to corporate life, Thomas decided to use his skill of communicating complex subject matter (comes with the territory of being in medical sales) to help others transform their lives, too. He started a YouTube channel to explain, in an accessible, compelling way, the biochemistry of the modalities that revitalized his life, confident that when people understood how these strategies work with their bodies, they would be empowered to try them for themselves. The YouTube channel surpassed one million subscribers within two years and now sits at close to 2.7 million subscribers and more than fifteen million views per month. Thomas remains committed to a nondogmatic approach to wellness and is passionate about sharing the latest research on how the human body functions to encourage everyone to find what works best for their unique biochemistry and optimize their life.

He has appeared in *Men's Health*, *Men's Fitness*, *Muscle & Fitness*, *Muscle & Performance*, and *Bodybuilding.com*, among other outlets.

Thomas lives with his wife, two young children, three dogs, and one trusty steed (their horse), near the central coast of California.

Additional Resources

For resources to support your intermittent fasting lifestyle, visit FastingIsEasy.com.

Notes

Introduction

1. Benefits of Fasting." *Obesity* 26 (2018): 254–268. doi:10.1002/oby.22065; de Cabo, Rafael and Mark P. Mattson. "Effects of Intermittent Fasting on Health, Aging, and Disease." *The New England Journal of Medicine* 381, no. 26 (2019): 2541–2551. doi:10.1056/NEJMra1905136.

2. Moro, Tatiana, et al. "Effects of Eight Weeks of Time-Restricted Feeding (16/8) on Basal Metabolism, Maximal Strength, Body Composition, Inflammation, and Cardiovascular Risk Factors in Resistance-Trained Males." *Journal of Translational Medicine* 14, no. 1 (2016): 290. doi:10.1186/s12967-016-1044-0; Varady, Krista A., et al. "Alternate-Day Fasting for Weight Loss in Normal Weight and Overweight Subjects: A Randomized Controlled Trial." *Nutrition Journal* 12, no. 1 (2013): 146. doi:10.1186/1475-2891-12-146.

3. Harvie, M.N., et al. "The Effects of Intermittent or Continuous Energy Restriction on Weight Loss and Metabolic Disease Risk Markers: A Randomized Trial in Young Overweight Women." *International Journal of Obesity* 35, no. 5 (2011): 714–27. doi:10.1038/ijo.2010.171.

4. Jordan, Stefan, et al. "Dietary Intake Regulates the Circulating Inflammatory Monocyte Pool." *Cell* 178, no. 5 (2019): 1102–1114.e17. doi:10.1016/j.cell.2019.07.050.

5. Mihaylova, Maria M., et al. "Fasting Activates Fatty Acid Oxidation to Enhance Intestinal Stem Cell Function During Homeostasis and Aging." *Cell Stem Cell* 22, no. 5 (2018): P769–778. doi:10.1016/j.stem.2018.04.001.

6. Mujica-Parodi, Lilianne R., et al. "Diet Modulates Brain Network Stability, a Biomarker for Brain Aging, in Young Adults." *Proceedings of the National Academy of Sciences* 117, no. 11 (2020): 6170–6177 .doi:10.1073/pnas.1913042117.

7. Marin, Traci, et al. "AMPK Promotes Mitochondrial Biogenesis and Function by Phosphorylating the Epigenetic Factors DNMT1, RBBP7, and HAT1." *Science Signaling* 10, no. 464 (2017): eaaf7478. doi:10.1126/scisignal.aaf7478.

8. Morris, Brian J., et al. "FOXO3: A Major Gene for Human Longevity—A Mini-Review." *Gerontology* 61, no. 6 (2015): 515–25. doi:10.1159/000375235.

9. Jamshed, Humaira, et al. "Early Time-Restricted Feeding Improves 24-Hour Glucose Levels and Affects Markers of the Circadian Clock, Aging, and Autophagy in Humans." *Nutrients* 11, no. 6 (2019): 1234. doi:10.3390/nu11061234.

Chapter 1: What Is Intermittent Fasting?

1. Anton, S.D., et al. "Flipping the Metabolic Switch: Understanding and Applying the Health Benefits of Fasting." *Obesity* 26 (2018): 254–268. doi:10.1002/oby.22065; de Cabo, Rafael and Mark P. Mattson. "Effects of Intermittent Fasting on Health, Aging, and Disease." *The New England Journal of Medicine* 381, no. 26 (2019): 2541–2551. doi:10.1056/NEJMra1905136.

2. Herzig, Sébastien and Reuben J. Shaw. "AMPK: Guardian of Metabolism and Mitochondrial Homeostasis." *Nature Reviews. Molecular Cell Biology* 19, no. 2 (2018): 121–135. doi:10.1038/nrm.2017.95.

3. Sztalryd, C. and F.B. Kraemer. "Regulation of Hormone-Sensitive Lipase During Fasting." *The American Journal of Physiology* 266, no. 2 Pt 1 (1994): E179–85. doi:10.1152/ajpendo.1994.266.2.E179.

4. Nørrelund, Helene, et al. "The Protein-Retaining Effects of Growth Hormone During Fasting Involve Inhibition of Muscle-Protein Breakdown." *Diabetes* 50, no. 1 (2001) 96–104. doi:10.2337/diabetes.50.1.96; Moller, Louise, et al. "Impact of Growth Hormone Receptor Blockade on Substrate Metabolism During Fasting in Healthy Subjects." *The Journal of Clinical Endocrinology & Metabolism* 94, no. 11 (2009): 4524–4532. doi:10.1210/jc.2009-0381.

5. Ottosson, M., et al. "The Effects of Cortisol on the Regulation of Lipoprotein Lipase Activity in Human Adipose Tissue." *The Journal of Clinical Endocrinology & Metabolism* 79, no. 3 (1994): 820–5. doi:10.1210/jcem.79.3.8077367.

6. Bergendahl, M., et al. "Short-Term Fasting Suppresses Leptin and (Conversely) Activates Disorderly Growth Hormone Secretion in Midluteal Phase Women—A Clinical Research Center Study." *The Journal of Clinical Endocrinology & Metabolism* 84, no. 3 (1999): 883–894. doi:10.1210/jcem.84.3.5536; Bergendahl, M., et al. "Fasting as a Metabolic Stress Paradigm Selectively Amplifies Cortisol Secretory Burst Mass and Delays the Time of Maximal Nyctohemeral Cortisol Concentrations in Healthy Men." *The Journal of Clinical Endocrinology & Metabolism* 81, no.2 (1996): 692–9.

7. Remelli, Francesca, et al. "Vitamin D Deficiency and Sarcopenia in Older Persons." *Nutrients* 11, no. 12 (2019): 2861. doi:10.3390/nu11122861; Garrido-Maraver, Juan, et al. "Clinical Applications of Coenzyme Q10." *Frontiers in Bioscience* (Landmark Edition) 19 (2014): 619–33. doi:10.2741/4231.

8. Harvie, M.N., et al. "The Effects of Intermittent or Continuous Energy Restriction on Weight Loss and Metabolic Disease Risk Markers: A Randomized Trial in Young Overweight Women." *International Journal of Obesity* 35, no. 5 (2011): 714–27. doi:10.1038/ijo.2010.171.

9. Moro, Tatiana, et al. "Effects of Eight Weeks of Time-Restricted Feeding (16/8) on Basal Metabolism, Maximal Strength, Body Composition, Inflammation, and Cardiovascular Risk Factors in Resistance-Trained Males." *Journal of Translational Medicine* 14, no. 1 (2016): 290. doi:10.1186/s12967-016-1044-0.

10. Vendelbo, Mikkel Holm, et al. "Fasting Increases Human Skeletal Muscle Net Phenylalanine Release and This Is Associated with Decreased mTOR Signaling." *PLOS One* 9, no. 7 (2014): e102031. doi:10.1371/journal.pone.0102031.

11. Hartman, M.L., et al. "Augmented Growth Hormone (GH) Secretory Burst Frequency and Amplitude Mediate Enhanced GH Secretion During a Two-Day Fast in Normal Men." *The Journal of Clinical Endocrinology & Metabolism* 74, no. 4 (1992): 757–65. doi:10.1210/jcem.74.4.1548337; Ho, K.Y., et al. "Fasting Enhances Growth Hormone Secretion and Amplifies the Complex Rhythms of Growth Hormone Secretion in Man." *The Journal of Clinical Investigation* 81, no. 4 (1988): 968–75. doi:10.1172/JCI113450.

12. Nørrelund, Helene, et al. "The Protein-Retaining Effects of Growth Hormone During Fasting Involve Inhibition of Muscle-Protein Breakdown." *Diabetes* 50, no. 1 (2001): 96–104. doi:10.2337/diabetes.50.1.96.

13. Nair, K.S., et al. "Effect of Beta-Hydroxybutyrate on Whole-Body Leucine Kinetics and Fractional Mixed Skeletal Muscle Protein Synthesis in Humans." *The Journal of Clinical Investigation* 82, no. 1 (1988): 198–205. doi:10.1172/JCI113570.

14. Heilbronn, Leonie K., et al. "Alternate-Day Fasting in Nonobese Subjects: Effects on Body Weight, Body Composition, and Energy Metabolism." *The American Journal of Clinical Nutrition* 81, no. 1 (2005): 69–73 .doi:10.1093/ajcn/81.1.69.

15. Webber J. and I.A. Macdonald. "The Cardiovascular, Metabolic, and Hormonal Changes Accompanying Acute Starvation in Men and Women." *British Journal of Nutrition* 71, no. 3 (1994): 437–47. doi:10.1079/bjn19940150.

16. Zauner, C., et al. "Resting Energy Expenditure in Short-Term Starvation Is Increased as a Result of an Increase in Serum Norepinephrine." *The American Journal of Clinical Nutrition* 71, no. 6 (2000): 1511–5. doi:10.1093/ajcn/71.6.1511.

17. Zauner, C., et al. "Resting Energy Expenditure in Short-Term Starvation Is Increased as a Result of an Increase in Serum Norepinephrine." *The American Journal of Clinical Nutrition* 71, no. 6 (2000): 1511–5. doi:10.1093/ajcn/71.6.1511.

18. Kumar, Sushil and Gurcharan Kaur. "Intermittent Fasting Dietary Restriction Regimen Negatively Influences Reproduction in Young Rats: A Study of Hypothalamo-Hypophysial-Gonadal Axis." *PLOS One* 8, no. 1 (2013): e52416. doi:10.1371/journal.pone.0052416.

19. Berga, Sarah L., et al. "Endocrine and Chronobiological Effects of Fasting in Women." *Reproductive Endocrinology* 75, no. 5 (2001): 926–932. doi:10.1016/S0015-0282(01)01686-7; Soules, M.R., et al. "Short-Term Fasting in Normal Women: Absence of Effects on Gonadotrophin Secretion and the Menstrual Cycle." *Clinical Endocrinology* 40, no. 6 (1994): 725–31. doi:10.1111/j.1365-2265.1994.tb02505.x.

20. O'Sullivan, A.J. "Does Oestrogen Allow Women to Store Fat More Efficiently? A Biological Advantage for Fertility and Gestation." *Obesity Reviews* 10, no. 2 (2009): 168–77. doi:10.1111/j.1467-789X.2008.00539.x.

21. Sztalryd, C. and F.B. Kraemer. "Regulation of Hormone-Sensitive Lipase During Fasting." *The American Journal of Physiology* 266, no. 2 Pt 1 (1994): E179–85. doi:10.1152/ajpendo.1994.266.2.E179.

22. Schmidt, Stacy L., et al. "Adrenergic Control of Lipolysis in Women Compared with Men." *Journal of Applied Physiology* 117, no. 9 (2014): 1008–1019. doi:10.1152/japplphysiol.00003.2014.

23. Tarnopolsky, M.A. "Sex Differences in Exercise Metabolism and the Role of 17-Beta Estradiol." *Medicine and Science in Sports and Exercise* 40, no. 4 (2008): 648–54. doi:10.1249/MSS.0b013e31816212ff.

24. Fliers, Eric, et al. "Beyond the Fixed Setpoint of the Hypothalamus-Pituitary-Thyroid Axis." *European Journal of Endocrinology* 171, no. 5 (2014): R197–208. doi:10.1530/EJE-14-0285; Boelen, A., et al. "Fasting-Induced Changes in the Hypothalamus-Pituitary-Thyroid Axis." *Thyroid* 18, no. 2 (2008): 123–129. doi:10.1089/thy.2007.0253.

25. Seimon, Radhika V., et al. "Do Intermittent Diets Provide Physiological Benefits Over Continuous Diets for Weight Loss? A Systematic Review of Clinical Trials." *Molecular and Cellular Endocrinology* 418, no. 2 (2015): 153–172. doi:10.1016/j.mce.2015.09.014.

26. Li, Guolin, et al. "Intermittent Fasting Promotes White Adipose Browning and Decreases Obesity by Shaping the Gut Microbiota." *Cell Metabolism* 26, no. 4 (2017): 672–-685.e4. doi:10.1016/j.cmet.2017.08.019.

27. Moro, Tatiana, et al. "Effects of Eight Weeks of Time-Restricted Feeding (16/8) on Basal Metabolism, Maximal Strength, Body Composition, Inflammation, and Cardiovascular Risk Factors in Resistance-Trained Males." *Journal of Translational Medicine* 14, no. 1 (2016): 290. doi:10.1186/s12967-016-1044-0.

28. Balasse, E.O. "Kinetics of Ketone Body Metabolism in Fasting Humans." *Metabolism* 28, no. 1 (1979): 41–50. doi:10.1016/0026-0495(79)90166-5.

29. Kim, K.H., et al. "Intermittent Fasting Promotes Adipose Thermogenesis and Metabolic Homeostasis via VEGF-mediated Alternative Activation of Macrophage." *Cell Research* 27 (2017): 1309–1326. doi:10.1038/cr.2017.126.

30. Sidossis, Labros and Shingo Kajimura. "Brown and Beige Fat in Humans: Thermogenic Adipocytes that Control Energy and Glucose Homeostasis." *The Journal of Clinical Investigation* 125, no. 2 (2015): 478–86. doi:10.1172/JCI78362; Cypess, Aaron M. and C. Ronald Kahn. "Brown Fat as a Therapy for Obesity and Diabetes." *Current Opinion in Endocrinology, Diabetes, and Obesity* 17, no. 2 (2010): 143–9. doi:10.1097/MED.0b013e328337a81f.

31. Madjd, Ameneh, et al. "Effects of Consuming Later Evening Meal vs. Earlier Evening Meal on Weight Loss During a Weight Loss Diet: A Randomised Clinical Trial." *British Journal of Nutrition* (2020): 1–9. doi:10.1017/S0007114520004456.

32. Ravussin, Eric, et al. "Early Time-Restricted Feeding Reduces Appetite and Increases Fat Oxidation but Does Not Affect Energy Expenditure in Humans." *Obesity* 27, no. 8 (2019): 1244. doi:10.1002/oby.22518.

33. Müller, James Manfred, et al. "Metabolic Adaptation to Caloric Restriction and Subsequent Refeeding: The Minnesota Starvation Experiment Revisited." *The American Journal of Clinical Nutrition* 102, no. 4 (2015): 807–19. doi:10.3945/ajcn.115.109173.

Chapter 2: Optimize Your Body

1. Sztalryd, C. and F.B. Kraemer. "Regulation of Hormone-Sensitive Lipase During Fasting." *The American Journal of Physiology* 266, no. 2 Pt 1 (1994): E179–85. doi:10.1152/ajpendo.1994.266.2.E179.

2. Harvie, M.N., et al. "The Effects of Intermittent or Continuous Energy Restriction on Weight Loss and Metabolic Disease Risk Markers: A Randomized Trial in Young Overweight Women." *International Journal of Obesity* 35, no. 5 (2011): 714–27. doi:10.1038/ijo.2010.171.

3. Habets, Daphna D.J., et al. "Crucial Role for LKB1 to AMPKalpha2 Axis in the Regulation of CD36-mediated Long-Chain Fatty Acid Uptake into Cardiomyocytes." *Biochimica et Biophysica Acta* 1791, no. 3 (2009): 212–9. doi:10.1016/j.bbalip.2008.12.009.

4. Marin, Traci L., et al. "AMPK Promotes Mitochondrial Biogenesis and Function by Phosphorylating the Epigenetic Factors DNMT1, RBBP7, and HAT1." *Science Signaling* 10, no. 464 (2017): eaaf7478. doi:10.1126/scisignal.aaf7478.

5. Ding, H., et al. "Fasting Induces a Subcutaneous-to-Visceral Fat Switch Mediated by MicroRNA-149-3p and Suppression of PRDM16." *Nature Communications* 7 (2016): 11533. doi:10.1038/ncomms11533.

6. Kim, K.H., et al. "Intermittent Fasting Promotes Adipose Thermogenesis and Metabolic Homeostasis via VEGF-Mediated Alternative Activation of Macrophage." *Cell Research* 27 (2017): 1309–1326. doi:10.1038/cr.2017.126.

7. Moro, Tatiana, et al. "Effects of Eight Weeks of Time-Restricted Feeding (16/8) on Basal Metabolism, Maximal Strength, Body Composition, Inflammation, and Cardiovascular Risk Factors in Resistance-Trained Males." *Journal of Translational Medicine* 14, no. 1 (2016): 290. doi:10.1186/s12967-016-1044-0.

8. Lee, David E., et al. "Autophagy as a Therapeutic Target to Enhance Aged Muscle Regeneration." *Cells* 8, no. 2 (2019): 183. doi:10.3390/cells8020183; Tang, Ann H., et al. "Induction of Autophagy Supports the Bioenergetic Demands of Quiescent Muscle Stem Cell Activation." *The EMBO Journal* 33, no. 23 (2014): 2782–97. doi:10.15252/embj.201488278.

9. Yoon, Mee-Sup. "The Role of Mammalian Target of Rapamycin (mTOR) in Insulin Signaling." *Nutrients* 9, no. 11 (2017): 1176. doi:10.3390/nu9111176.

10. Deldicque, L., et al. "Increased p70s6k Phosphorylation During Intake of a Protein–Carbohydrate Drink Following Resistance Exercise in the Fasted State." *European Journal of Applied Physiology* 108 (2010): 791–800. doi:10.1007/s00421-009-1289-x.

11. Morris, Brian J., et al. "FOXO3: A Major Gene for Human Longevity—A Mini-Review." *Gerontology* 61, no. 6 (2015): 515–25. doi:10.1159/000375235.

12. Pawlak, Michal, et al. "Molecular Mechanism of PPAR-α Action and Its Impact on Lipid Metabolism, Inflammation and Fibrosis in Non-Alcoholic Fatty Liver Disease." *Journal of Hepatology* 62, no. 3 (2015): 720–33. doi:10.1016/j.jhep.2014.10.039.

13. McCormack, Shana, et al. "Pharmacologic Targeting of Sirtuin and PPAR Signaling Improves Longevity and Mitochondrial Physiology in Respiratory Chain Complex I Mutant Caenorhabditis Elegans." *Mitochondrion* 22 (2015): 45–59. doi:10.1016/j.mito.2015.02.005.

14. Vitale, Giovanni, et al. "ROLE of IGF-1 System in the Modulation of Longevity: Controversies and New Insights from a Centenarian's Perspective." *Frontiers in Endocrinology* 10 (2019): 27. doi:10.3389/fendo.2019.00027.

15. Bagherniya, Mohammad, et al. "The Effect of Fasting or Calorie Restriction on Autophagy Induction: A Review of the Literature." *Ageing Research Reviews* 47 (2018): 183–197. doi:10.1016/j.arr.2018.08.004.

16. Glick, Danielle, et al. "Autophagy: Cellular and Molecular Mechanisms." *The Journal of Pathology* 221, no. 1 (2010): 3–12. doi:10.1002/path.2697.

17. Zoncu, R., et al. "mTOR: From Growth Signal Integration to Cancer, Diabetes, and Aging." *National Review Molecular Cell Biology* 12 (2011): 21–35. doi:10.1038/nrm3025.

18. Mihaylove, Maria M., et al. "Fasting Activates Fatty Acid Oxidation to Enhance Intestinal Stem Cell Function During Homeostasis and Aging." *Cell Stem Cell* 22, no. 5 (2018): P769–778. doi:10.1016/j.stem.2018.04.001.

19. Ramunas, J., et al. "Transient Delivery of Modified mRNA Encoding TERT Rapidly Extends Telomeres in Human Cells." *The FASEB Journal* 29 (2015): 1930–1939. doi:10.1096/fj.14-259531.

20. Vera, Elsa, et al. "Telomerase Reverse Transcriptase Synergizes with Calorie Restriction to Increase Health Span and Extend Mouse Longevity." *PLOS One* 8, no. 1 (2013): e53760. doi:10.1371/journal.pone.0053760.

21. Aguilar, M. "Prevalence of the Metabolic Syndrome in the United States, 2003–2012." *JAMA* 313, no. 19 (2015): 1973–1974. doi:10.1001/jama.2015.4260.

22. Sutton, Elizabeth F., et al. "Early Time-Restricted Feeding Improves Insulin Sensitivity, Blood Pressure, and Oxidative Stress Even without Weight Loss in Men with Prediabetes." *Cell Metabolism* 27, no. 6 (2018): 1212–1221.e3. doi:10.1016/j.cmet.2018.04.010.

23. Harvie, M.N., et al. "The Effects of Intermittent or Continuous Energy Restriction on Weight Loss and Metabolic Disease Risk Markers: A Randomized Trial in Young Overweight Women." *International Journal of Obesity* 35, no. 5 (2011): 714–27. doi:10.1038/ijo.2010.171.

24. Hardie, D., et al. "AMPK: A Nutrient and Energy Sensor that Maintains Energy Homeostasis." *Nature Reviews Molecular Cell Biology* 13 (2012): 251–262. doi:10.1038/nrm3311.

25. Furman, D., et al. "Chronic Inflammation in the Etiology of Disease Across the Life Span." *Nature Medicine* 25 (2019): 1822–1832. doi:10.1038/s41591-019-0675-0.

26. National Institute of Diabetes and Digestive and Kidney Diseases. "Nonalcoholic Fatty Liver Disease and NASH." niddk.nih.gov/health-information/liver-disease/nafld-nash/all-content.

27. Li, Yu, et al. "AMPK Phosphorylates and Inhibits SREBP Activity to Attenuate Hepatic Steatosis and Atherosclerosis in Diet-Induced Insulin-Resistant Mice." *Cell Metabolism* 13, no. 4 (2011): 376–388. doi:10.1016/j.cmet.2011.03.009.

28. Hatchwell, Luke, et al. "Multi-omics Analysis of the Intermittent Fasting Response in Mice Identifies an Unexpected Role for HNF4α." *Cell Reports* 30, no. 10 (2020): 3566. doi:10.1016/j.celrep.2020.02.051.

29. Wegman, Martin P., et al. "Practicality of Intermittent Fasting in Humans and Its Effect on Oxidative Stress and Genes Related to Aging and Metabolism." *Rejuvenation Research* 18, no. 2 (2015): 162–72. doi:10.1089/rej.2014.1624.

30. Youm, Y.H., et al. "The Ketone Metabolite β-hydroxybutyrate Blocks NLRP3 Inflammasome–Mediated Inflammatory Disease." *Nature Medicine* 21 (2015): 263–269. doi:10.1038/nm.3804.

31. Jordan, Stefan, et al. "Dietary Intake Regulates the Circulating Inflammatory Monocyte Pool." *Cell* 178, no. 5 (2019): 1102–1114.e17. doi:10.1016/j.cell.2019.07.050.

32. Moro, Tatiana, et al. "Effects of Eight Weeks of Time-Restricted Feeding (16/8) on Basal Metabolism, Maximal Strength, Body Composition, Inflammation, and Cardiovascular Risk Factors in Resistance-Trained Males." *Journal of Translational Medicine* 14, no. 1 (2016): 290. doi:10.1186/s12967-016-1044-0.

33. Sutton, Elizabeth F., et al. "Early Time-Restricted Feeding Improves Insulin Sensitivity, Blood Pressure, and Oxidative Stress Even Without Weight Loss in Men with Prediabetes." *Cell Metabolism* 27, no. 6 (2018): 1212–1221.e3. doi:10.1016/j.cmet.2018.04.010.

34. Hardie, D.G., et al. "Regulation of Fatty Acid Synthesis and Oxidation by the AMP-Activated Protein Kinase." *Biochemical Society Transactions* 30, no. 6 (2002): 1064–1070. doi:10.1042/bst0301064.

35. Bhutani, Surabhi, et al. "Improvements in Coronary Heart Disease Risk Indicators by Alternate-Day Fasting Involve Adipose Tissue Modulations." *Obesity* 18, no. 11 (2010): 2152–9. doi:10.1038/oby.2010.54.

36. Carling, D., et al. "Purification and Characterization of the AMP-Activated Protein Kinase. Copurification of Acetyl-CoA Carboxylase Kinase and 3-Hydroxy-3-Methylglutaryl-CoA Reductase Kinase Activities." *European Journal of Biochemistry* 186 (1989): 129–36. doi:10.1111/j.1432-1033.1989.tb15186.x.

37. Bhutani, Surabhi, et al. "Improvements in Coronary Heart Disease Risk Indicators by Alternate-Day Fasting Involve Adipose Tissue Modulations." *Obesity* 18, no. 11 (2010): 2152–9. doi:10.1038/oby.2010.54.

38. Buccelletti, E., et al. "Heart Rate Variability and Myocardial Infarction: Systematic Literature Review and Metanalysis." *European Review for Medical and Pharmacological Sciences* 13, no. 4 (2009): 299–307. PMID:19694345.

39. Cansel, Mehmet, et al. "The Effects of Ramadan Fasting on Heart Rate Variability in Healthy Individuals: A Prospective Study." *Anadolu Kardiyoloji Dergisi* (*The Anatolian Journal of Cardiology*) 14, no. 5 (2014): 413–6. doi:10.5152/akd.2014.5108.

40. Han, Young-min, et al. "β-Hydroxybutyrate Prevents Vascular Senescence Through hnRNP A1-Mediated Upregulation of Oct4." *Molecular Cell* 71, no. 6 (2018): 1064–1078.e5. doi:10.1016/j.molcel.2018.07.036.

41. Jordan, Stefan, et al. "Dietary Intake Regulates the Circulating Inflammatory Monocyte Pool." *Cell* 178, no. 5 (2019): 1102–1114.e17. doi:10.1016/j.cell.2019.07.050; Collins, Nicholas, et al. "The Bone Marrow Protects and Optimizes Immunological Memory During Dietary Restriction." *Cell* 178, no. 5 (2019): 1088–1101.e15. doi:10.1016/j.cell.2019.07.049.

42. Vighi, G., et al. "Allergy and the Gastrointestinal System." *Clinical and Experimental Immunology* 153, Suppl 1 (2008): 3–6. doi:10.1111/j.1365-2249.2008.03713.x.

43. Cheng, Chia-Wei, et al. "Prolonged Fasting Reduces IGF-1/PKA to Promote Hematopoietic-Stem-Cell-Based Regeneration and Reverse Immunosuppression." *Cell Stem Cell* 14, no. 6 (2014): 810–23. doi:10.1016/j.stem.2014.04.014.

44. Collins, Nicholas, et al. "The Bone Marrow Protects and Optimizes Immunological Memory During Dietary Restriction." *Cell* 178, no. 5 (2019): 1088–1101.e15. doi:10.1016/j.cell.2019.07.049.

45. Mihaylova, Maria M., et al. "Fasting Activates Fatty Acid Oxidation to Enhance Intestinal Stem Cell Function During Homeostasis and Aging." *Cell Stem Cell* 22, no. 5 (2018): P769–778. doi:10.1016/j.stem.2018.04.001.

46. Li, Guolin, et al. "Intermittent Fasting Promotes White Adipose Browning and Decreases Obesity by Shaping the Gut Microbiota." *Cell Metabolism* 26, no. 4 (2017): 672–685.e4. doi:10.1016/j.cmet.2017.08.019.

47. Catanzaro, Jason R., et al. "IgA-deficient Humans Exhibit Gut Microbiota Dysbiosis Despite Production of Compensatory IgM." *Scientific Reports* 9, no. 13574 (2019). doi:10.1101/446724.

48. Godínez Victoria, M., et al. "Intermittent Fasting Promotes Bacterial Clearance and Intestinal IgA Production in *Salmonella typhimurium* Infected Mice." *Scandinavian Journal of Immunology* 79 (2014): 315–324. doi:10.1111/sji.12163.

49. Mihaylova, Maria M., et al. "Fasting Activates Fatty Acid Oxidation to Enhance Intestinal Stem Cell Function During Homeostasis and Aging." *Cell Stem Cell* 22, no. 5 (2018): P769–778. doi:10.1016/j.stem.2018.04.001.

50. Sato, K., et al. "Insulin, Ketone Bodies, and Mitochondrial Energy Transduction." *The FASEB Journal* 9 (1995): 651–658. doi:10.1096/fasebj.9.8.7768357.

51. Marin, Traci, et al. "AMPK Promotes Mitochondrial Biogenesis and Function by Phosphorylating the Epigenetic Factors DNMT1, RBBP7, and HAT1." *Science Signaling* 10, no. 464 (2017): eaaf7478. doi:10.1126/scisignal.aaf7478.

52. Sato, Kashiwaya K., et al. "Insulin, Ketone Bodies, and Mitochondrial Energy Transduction." *The FASEB Journal* 9 (1995): 651–658. doi:10.1096/fasebj.9.8.7768357.

53. Michalsen, A., et al. "Effects of Short-Term Modified Fasting on Sleep Patterns and Daytime Vigilance in Non-Obese Subjects: Results of a Pilot Study." *Annals of Nutrition and Metabolism* 47 (2003): 194–200. doi:10.1159/000070485.

54. Kvietys, P.R. "Chapter 5: Postprandial Hyperemia." in *The Gastrointestinal Circulation*. San Rafael, CA: Morgan & Claypool Life Sciences, 2010. Available from: ncbi.nlm.nih.gov/books/NBK53094/.

Chapter 3: Optimize Your Mind

1. Singh, Rumani, et al. "Late-Onset Intermittent Fasting Dietary Restriction as a Potential Intervention to Retard Age-Associated Brain Function Impairments in Male Rats." *Age* 34, no. 4 (2012): 917–33. doi:10.1007/s11357-011-9289-2.

2. Fontán-Lozano, Angela, et al. "Caloric Restriction Increases Learning Consolidation and Facilitates Synaptic Plasticity Through Mechanisms Dependent on NR2B Subunits of the NMDA Receptor." *The Journal of Neuroscience* 27, no. 38 (2007): 10185–95. doi:10.1523/JNEUROSCI.2757-07.2007.

3. Green, M.W., et al. "Lack of Effect of Short-Term Fasting on Cognitive Function." *Journal of Psychiatric Research* 29, no. 3 (1995): 245–53. doi:10.1016/0022-3956(95)00009-t.

4. Lieberman, Harris R., et al. "A Double-Blind, Placebo-Controlled Test of 2 D of Calorie Deprivation: Effects on Cognition, Activity, Sleep, and Interstitial Glucose Concentrations." *The American Journal of Clinical Nutrition* 88, no. 3 (2008): 667–76. doi:10.1093/ajcn/88.3.667.

5. Mattson, Mark P., et al. "Meal Size and Frequency Affect Neuronal Plasticity and Vulnerability to Disease: Cellular and Molecular Mechanisms." *Journal of Neurochemistry* 84, no. 3 (2003): 417–31. doi:10.1046/j.1471-4159.2003.01586.x; Mattson, Mark P. "Energy Intake, Meal Frequency, and Health: A Neurobiological Perspective." *Annual Review of Nutrition* 25 (2005): 237–60. doi:10.1146/annurev.nutr.25.050304.092526.

6. Burkhalter, Julia, et al. "Brain-Derived Neurotrophic Factor Stimulates Energy Metabolism in Developing Cortical Neurons." *The Journal of Neuroscience* 23, no. 23 (2003): 8212–20. doi:10.1523/JNEUROSCI.23-23-08212.2003.

7. Halagappa, Veerendra Kumar Madala, et al. "Intermittent Fasting and Caloric Restriction Ameliorate Age-Related Behavioral Deficits in the Triple-Transgenic Mouse Model of Alzheimer's Disease." *Neurobiology of Disease* 26, no. 1 (2007): 212–20. doi:10.1016/j.nbd.2006.12.019; Mattson, Mark P., et al. "Impact of Intermittent Fasting on Health and Disease Processes." *Ageing Research Reviews* 39 (2017): 46–58. doi:10.1016/j.arr.2016.10.005.

8. Erickson, Kirk I., et al. "Brain-Derived Neurotrophic Factor Is Associated with Age-Related Decline in Hippocampal Volume." *The Journal of Neuroscience* 30, no. 15 (2010): 5368-75. doi:10.1523/JNEUROSCI.6251-09.2010.

9. Kim, Sang Woo, et al. "Ketone Beta-Hydroxybutyrate Up-Regulates BDNF Expression Through NF-κB as an Adaptive Response Against ROS, Which May Improve Neuronal Bioenergetics and Enhance Neuroprotection." *Neurology* 88 (2017): P3.090; Mattson, Mark P., et al. "Impact of Intermittent Fasting on Health and Disease Processes." *Ageing Research Reviews* 39 (2017): 46–58. doi:10.1016/j.arr.2016.10.005.

10. Mujica-Parodi, Lilianne R., et al. "Diet Modulates Brain Network Stability, a Biomarker for Brain Aging, in Young Adults." *Proceedings of the National Academy of Sciences* 117, no. 11 (2020): 6170–6177. doi:10.1073/pnas.1913042117.

11. Noh, Hae Sook, et al. "A cDNA Microarray Analysis of Gene Expression Profiles in Rat Hippocampus Following a Ketogenic Diet." *Molecular Brain Research* 129, nos. 1–2 (2004): 80–7. doi:10.1016/j.molbrainres.2004.06.020.

12. Maalouf, M., et al. "Ketones Inhibit Mitochondrial Production of Reactive Oxygen Species Production Following Glutamate Excitotoxicity by Increasing NADH Oxidation." *Neuroscience* 145, no. 1 (2007): 256–264. doi:10.1016/j.neuroscience.2006.11.065.

13. Institute for Neurodegenerative Disease. https://ind.ucsf.edu/supporting-our-work/extent-problem; Parkinson's Foundation. Parkinson.org/Understanding-Parkinsons/Statistics.

14. Nilsson, Per, et al. "Aβ Secretion and Plaque Formation Depend on Autophagy." *Cell Reports* 5, no. 1 (2013): 61–9. doi:10.1016/j.celrep.2013.08.042.

15. Vasconcelos, Andrea Rodrigues, et al. "Effects of Intermittent Fasting on Age-Related Changes on Na,K-ATPase Activity and Oxidative Status Induced by Lipopolysaccharide in Rat Hippocampus." *Neurobiology of Aging* 36, no. 5 (2015): 1914–23. doi:10.1016/j.neurobiolaging.2015.02.020.

16. de la Monte, Suzanne M. and Jack R. Wands. "Alzheimer's Disease Is Type 3 Diabetes-Evidence Reviewed." *Journal of Diabetes Science and Technology* 2, no. 6 (2008): 1101–13. doi:10.1177/193229680800200619; Norwitz, Nicholas G., et al. "Multi-Loop Model of Alzheimer Disease: An Integrated Perspective on the Wnt/GSK3β, α-Synuclein, and Type 3 Diabetes Hypotheses." *Frontiers in Aging Neuroscience* 11 (2019): 184. doi:10.3389/fnagi.2019.00184.

17. Hussin, N.M., et al. "Efficacy of Fasting and Calorie Restriction (FCR) on Mood and Depression Among Aging Men." *The Journal of Nutrition, Health & Aging* 17, no. 8 (2013): 674–80. doi:10.1007/s12603-013-0344-9.

18. Bastani, Abdolhossein, et al. "The Effects of Fasting During Ramadan on the Concentration of Serotonin, Dopamine, Brain-Derived Neurotrophic Factor and Nerve Growth Factor." *Neurology International* 9, no. 2 (2017): 7043. doi:10.4081/ni.2017.7043.

19. Towers, Albert E., et al. "Acute Fasting Inhibits Central Caspase-1 Activity Reducing Anxietylike Behavior and Increasing Novel Object and Object Location Recognition." *Metabolism: Clinical and Experimental* 71 (2017): 70–82. doi:10.1016/j.metabol.2017.03.005.

20. Lutas, Andrew and Gary Yellen. "The Ketogenic Diet: Metabolic Influences on Brain Excitability and Epilepsy." *Trends in Neurosciences* 36, no. 1 (2013): 32–40. doi:10.1016/j.tins.2012.11.005.

21. Carhart-Harris, R.L. and D.J. Nutt. "Serotonin and Brain Function: A Tale of Two Receptors." *Journal of Psychopharmacology* (Oxford, England) 31, no. 9 (2017): 1091–1120. doi:10.1177/0269881117725915.

Chapter 4: Your Fasting Window

1. Grygiel-Górniak, B. "Peroxisome Proliferator-Activated Receptors and Their Ligands: Nutritional and Clinical Implications—A Review." *Nutrition Journal* 13 (2014): 17. doi:10.1186/1475-2891-13-17.

2. Romon, M., et al. "Leptin Response to Carbohydrate or Fat Meal and Association with Subsequent Satiety and Energy Intake." *The American Journal of Physiology* 277, no. 5 (1999): E855–61. doi:10.1152/ajpendo.1999.277.5.E855.

3. Perry, Rachel J., et al. "Leptin Mediates a Glucose-Fatty Acid Cycle to Maintain Glucose Homeostasis in Starvation." *Cell* 172, nos. 1–2 (2018): P234–248. doi:10.1016/j.cell.2017.12.001.

4. St-Pierre, Valerie, et al. "Butyrate Is More Ketogenic than Leucine or Octanoate-Monoacylglycerol in Healthy Adult Humans." *Journal of Functional Foods* 32 (2017): 170–175. doi:10.1016/j.jff.2017.02.024; Hird, F.J. and R.H. Symons. "The Mechanism of Ketone-Body Formation from Butyrate in Rat Liver." *The Biochemical Journal* 84, no. 1 (1962): 212–6. doi:10.1042/bj0840212.

5. Wu, X. and J. Xu. "New Role of Hispidulin in Lipid Metabolism: PPAR-α Activator." *Lipids* 51 (2016): 1249–1257. doi:10.1007/s11745-016-4200-7; Mueller, Monika, et al. "Oregano: A Source for Peroxisome Proliferator-Activated Receptor γ Antagonists." *Journal of Agricultural and Food Chemistry* 56, no. 24 (2008): 11621–11630. doi:10.1021/jf802298w; Rigano, Daniela, et al. "The Potential of Natural Products for Targeting PPAR-α." *Acta Pharmaceutica Sinica B* 7, no. 4 (2017): 427–438. doi:10.1016/j.apsb.2017.05.005.

6. Klimek-Szczykutowicz, Marta, et al. "*Citrus limon* (Lemon) Phenomenon—A Review of the Chemistry, Pharmacological Properties, Applications in the Modern Pharmaceutical, Food, and Cosmetics Industries, and Biotechnological Studies." *Plants* 9, no. 1 (2020): 119. doi:10.3390/plants9010119.

7. Echeverri, Dario, et al. "Caffeine's Vascular Mechanisms of Action." *International Journal of Vascular Medicine* 2010 (2010): 834060. doi:10.1155/2010/834060.

8. Pietrocola, Federico, et al. "Coffee Induces Autophagy In Vivo." *Cell Cycle* 13, no. 12 (2014): 1987–94. doi:10.4161/cc.28929.

9. Rocha, A., et al. "Green Tea Extract Activates AMPK and Ameliorates White Adipose Tissue Metabolic Dysfunction Induced by Obesity." *European Journal of Nutrition* 55 (2016): 2231–2244. doi:10.1007/s00394-015-1033-8.

10. Lu, Hong, et al. "Enzymology of Methylation of Tea Catechins and Inhibition of Catechol-O-Methyltransferase by (-)-Epigallocatechin Gallate." *Drug Metabolism and Disposition: The Biological Fate of Chemicals* 31, no. 5 (2003): 572–9. doi:10.1124/dmd.31.5.572.

11. Asfar, Sami, et al. "Effect of Green Tea in the Prevention and Reversal of Fasting-Induced Intestinal Mucosal Damage." *Nutrition* 19, no. 6 (2003): 536–40. doi:10.1016/s0899-9007(02)01097-3.

12. Zhang, Yi, et al. "Leaves of *Lippia triphylla* Improve Hepatic Lipid Metabolism via Activating AMPK to Regulate Lipid Synthesis and Degradation." *Journal of Natural Medicines* 73, no. 4 (2019): 707–716. doi:10.1007/s11418-019-01316-5.

13. Weinsier, Roland L. "Fasting—A Review with Emphasis on the Electrolytes." *The American Journal of Medicine* 50, no. 2 (1971): P233–240.

14. Weinsier, Roland L. "Fasting—A Review with Emphasis on the Electrolytes." *The American Journal of Medicine* 50, no. 2 (1971): P233–240.

15. Drenick, Ernst J., et al. "Magnesium Depletion During Prolonged Fasting of Obese Males." *The Journal of Clinical Endocrinology & Metabolism* 29, no. 10 (1969): 1341–134. doi:10.1210/jcem-29-10-1341; Fisler, J.S., et al. "Calcium, Magnesium, and Phosphate Balances During Very Low Calorie Diets of Soy or Collagen Protein in Obese Men: Comparison to Total Fasting." *The American Journal of Clinical Nutrition* 40, no. 1 (1984): 14–25. doi:10.1093/ajcn/40.1.14.

16. Prielipp, R.C., et al. "Magnesium Inhibits the Hypertensive but Not the Cardiotonic Actions of Low-Dose Epinephrine." *Anesthesiology* 74, no. 6 (1991): 973–9. doi:10.1097/00000542-199106000-00002.

17. Wegman, Martin P., et al. "Practicality of Intermittent Fasting in Humans and Its Effect on Oxidative Stress and Genes Related to Aging and Metabolism." *Rejuvenation Research* 18, no. 2 (2015): 162–72. doi:10.1089/rej.2014.1624.

18. Sakakibara, Shoji, et al. "Acetic Acid Activates Hepatic AMPK and Reduces Hyperglycemia in Diabetic KK-A(y) Mice." *Biochemical and Biophysical Research Communications* 344, no. 2 (2006): 597–604. doi:10.1016/j.bbrc.2006.03.176.

19. Kondo, Tomoo, et al. "Acetic Acid Upregulates the Expression of Genes for Fatty Acid Oxidation Enzymes in Liver to Suppress Body Fat Accumulation." *Journal of Agriculture and Food Chemistry* 57, no. 13 (2009): 5982–5986. doi:10.1021/jf900470c.

20. Bjarnsholt, Thomas, et al. "Antibiofilm Properties of Acetic Acid." *Advances in Wound Care* 4, no. 7 (2015): 363–372. doi:10.1089/wound.2014.0554.

21. Suk, Sujin, et al. "Gingerenone A, a Polyphenol Present in Ginger, Suppresses Obesity and Adipose Tissue Inflammation in High-Fat Diet-Fed Mice." *Molecular Nutrition & Food Research* 61, no. 10 (2017). doi:10.1002/mnfr.201700139.

22. Iwasaki, Yusaku, et al. "A Nonpungent Component of Steamed Ginger—[10]-Shogaol—Increases Adrenaline Secretion via the Activation of TRPV1." *Nutritional Neuroscience* 9, nos. 3–4 (2006): 169–78. doi:10.1080/110284150600955164.

23. Townsend, Elizabeth A., et al. "Active Components of Ginger Potentiate β-agonist-induced Relaxation of Airway Smooth Muscle by Modulating Cytoskeletal Regulatory Proteins." *American Journal of Respiratory Cell and Molecular Biology* 50, no. 1 (2014): 115–24. doi:10.1165/rcmb.2013-0133OC.

24. Ludy, Mary-Jon, et al. "The Effects of Capsaicin and Capsiate on Energy Balance: Critical Review and Meta-Analyses of Studies in Humans." *Chemical Senses* 37, no. 2 (2012): 103–21. doi:10.1093/chemse/bjr100.

25. Wang, Chen, et al. "Downregulation of PI3K/Akt/mTOR Signaling Pathway in Curcumin-Induced Autophagy in APP/PS1 Double Transgenic Mice." *European Journal of Pharmacology* 740 (2014): 312–20. doi:10.1016/j.ejphar.2014.06.051; Shakeri, Abolfazl, et al. "Curcumin: A Naturally Occurring Autophagy Modulator." *Journal of Cellular Physiology* 234, no. 5 (2019): 5643–5654. doi:10.1002/jcp.27404.

26. Song, Ju-Xian, et al. "A Novel Curcumin Analog Binds to and Activates TFEB In Vitro and In Vivo Independent of MTOR Inhibition." *Autophagy* 12, no. 8 (2016): 1372–89. doi:10.1080/15548627.2016.1179404.

27. Hamidie, Ronald D. Ray, et al. "Curcumin Treatment Enhances the Effect of Exercise on Mitochondrial Biogenesis in Skeletal Muscle by Increasing cAMP Levels." *Metabolism* 64, no. 10 (2015): 1334–1347. doi:10.1016/j.metabol.2015.07.010.

28. Qin, Bolin, et al. "Cinnamon: Potential Role in the Prevention of Insulin Resistance, Metabolic Syndrome, and Type 2 Diabetes." *Journal of Diabetes Science and Technology* 4, no. 3 (2010): 685–93. doi:10.1177/193229681000400324; Jarvill-Taylor, K.J., et al. "A Hydroxychalcone Derived from Cinnamon Functions as a Mimetic for Insulin in 3T3-L1 Adipocytes." *Journal of the American College of Nutrition* 20, no. 4 (2001): 327–336. doi:10.1080/07315724.2001.10719053.

29. Ruiz-Ojeda, Francisco Javier, et al. "Effects of Sweeteners on the Gut Microbiota: A Review of Experimental Studies and Clinical Trials." *Advances in Nutrition* 10, no. 1 (2019): S31–S48. doi:10.1093/advances/nmy037; Abou-Donia, Mohamed B., et al. "Splenda Alters Gut Microflora and Increases Intestinal P-Glycoprotein and Cytochrome P-450 in Male Rats." *Journal of Toxicology and Environmental Health Part A* 71, no. 21 (2008): 1415–29. doi:10.1080/15287390802328630.

30. Wolever, Thomas M.S., et al. "Sugar Alcohols and Diabetes: A Review." *Canadian Journal of Diabetes* 26, no. 4 (2002): 356–362.

31. Noda, K., et al. "Serum Glucose and Insulin Levels and Erythritol Balance After Oral Administration of Erythritol in Healthy Subjects." *European Journal of Clinical Nutrition* 48, no. 4 (1994): 286–92. PMID:8039489.

32. Pereira, Amanda Gomes, et al. "Effects of Fluoride on Insulin Signaling and Bone Metabolism in Ovariectomized Rats." *Journal of Trace Elements in Medicine and Biology*. 39 (2017): 140–146. doi:10.1016/j.jtemb.2016.09.007.

33. Hobson, R.M., et al. "Effects of β-alanine Supplementation on Exercise Performance: A Meta-Analysis." *Amino Acids* 43, no. 1 (2012): 25–37. doi:10.1007/s00726-011-1200-z.

34. Doherty, M. and P.M. Smith. "Effects of Caffeine Ingestion on Rating of Perceived Exertion During and After Exercise: A Meta-Analysis." *Scandinavian Journal of Medicine & Science in Sports* 15 (2005): 69–78. doi:10.1111/j.1600-0838.2005.00445.x.

35. Wegman, Martin P., et al. "Practicality of Intermittent Fasting in Humans and Its Effect on Oxidative Stress and Genes Related to Aging and Metabolism." *Rejuvenation Research* 18, no. 2 (2015): 162–72. doi:10.1089/rej.2014.1624.

36. Kalogeropoulou, Dionysia, et al. "Leucine, When Ingested with Glucose, Synergistically Stimulates Insulin Secretion and Lowers Blood Glucose." *Metabolism: Clinical and Experimental* 57, no. 12 (2008): 1747–52. doi:10.1016/j.metabol.2008.09.001; Gran, Petra and David Cameron-Smith. "The Actions of Exogenous Leucine on mTOR Signaling and Amino Acid Transporters in Human Myotubes." *BMC Physiology* 11, no. 10 (2011). doi:10.1186/1472-6793-11-10.

37. De Bock, K., et al. "Effect of Training in the Fasted State on Metabolic Responses During Exercise with Carbohydrate Intake." *Journal of Applied Physiology* 104, no. 4 (2008): 1045–1055. doi:10.1152/japplphysiol.01195.2007.

38. Van Proeyen, Karen, et al. "Training in the Fasted State Improves Glucose Tolerance During Fat-Rich Diet." *The Journal of Physiology* 588, no. 21 (2010): 4289–302. doi:10.1113/jphysiol.2010.196493.

39. De Bock, K., et al. "Effect of Training in the Fasted State on Metabolic Responses During Exercise with Carbohydrate Intake." *Journal of Applied Physiology* 104, no. 4 (2008): 1045–1055. doi:10.1152/japplphysiol.01195.2007.

40. De Bock, K., et al. "Effect of Training in the Fasted State on Metabolic Responses During Exercise with Carbohydrate Intake." *Journal of Applied Physiology* 104, no. 4 (2008): 1045–1055. doi:10.1152/japplphysiol.01195.2007.

41. He, Congcong, et al. "Exercise Induces Autophagy in Peripheral Tissues and in the Brain." *Autophagy* 8, no. 10 (2012): 1548–51. doi:10.4161/auto.21327.

42. Sardeli, Amanda V., et al. "Resistance Training Prevents Muscle Loss Induced by Caloric Restriction in Obese Elderly Individuals: A Systematic Review and Meta-Analysis." *Nutrients* 10, no. 4 (2018): 423. doi:10.3390/nu10040423

43. Song, Z., et al. "Resistance Exercise Initiates Mechanistic Target of Rapamycin (mTOR) Translocation and Protein Complex Co-Localisation in Human Skeletal Muscle." *Scientific Reports* 7, no. 5028 (2017). doi:10.1038/s41598-017-05483-x.

44. Song, Z., et al. "Resistance Exercise Initiates Mechanistic Target of Rapamycin (mTOR) Translocation and Protein Complex Co-Localisation in Human Skeletal Muscle." *Scientific Reports* 7, no. 5028 (2017). doi:10.1038/s41598-017-05483-x.

45. Cramer, Holger, et al. "Yoga in Women with Abdominal Obesity, a Randomized Controlled Trial." *Deutsches Arzteblatt International* 113, no. 39 (2016): 645–652. doi:10.3238/arztebl.2016.0645; Neumark-Sztainer, Dianne, et al. "How Is the Practice of Yoga Related to Weight Status? Population-Based Findings from Project EAT-IV." *Journal of Physical Activity & Health* 14, no. 12 (2017): 905–912. doi:10.1123/jpah.2016-0608.

46. Boschmann, Michael, et al. "Water-Induced Thermogenesis." *The Journal of Clinical Endocrinology & Metabolism* 88, no. 12 (2003): 6015–9. doi:10.1210/jc.2003-030780.

47. Massolt, Elske T., et al. "Appetite Suppression Through Smelling of Dark Chocolate Correlates with Changes in Ghrelin in Young Women." *Regulatory Peptides* 161, nos. 1–3 (2010): 81–6. doi:10.1016/j.regpep.2010.01.005.

48. Mathern, Jocelyn R., et al. "Effect of Fenugreek Fiber on Satiety, Blood Glucose, and Insulin Response and Energy Intake in Obese Subjects." *Phytotherapy Research: PTR* 23, no. 11 (2009): 1543–8. doi:10.1002/ptr.2795.

49. Chevassus, Hugues, et al. "A Fenugreek Seed Extract Selectively Reduces Spontaneous Fat Consumption in Healthy Volunteers." *European Journal of Clinical Pharmacology* 65, no. 12 (2009): 1175–8. doi:10.1007/s00228-009-0733-5.

50. Kaats, Gilbert R., et al. "Konjac Glucomannan Dietary Supplementation Causes Significant Fat Loss in Compliant Overweight Adults." *Journal of the American College of Nutrition.* (2015): 1–7. doi:10.1080/07315724.2015.1009194.

51. Alkhatib, Ahmad and Roisin Atcheson. "Yerba Maté (*Ilex paraguariensis*) Metabolic, Satiety, and Mood State Effects at Rest and During Prolonged Exercise." *Nutrients* 9, no. 8 (2017): 882. doi.org/10.3390/nu9080882; Mansour, Muhammad S., et al. "Ginger Consumption Enhances the Thermic Effect of Food and Promotes Feelings of Satiety Without Affecting Metabolic and Hormonal Parameters in Overweight Men: A Pilot Study." *Metabolism: Clinical and Experimental* 61, no. 10 (2012): 1347–52. doi:10.1016/j.metabol.2012.03.016.

52. Ludy, Mary-Jon, et al. "The Effects of Capsaicin and Capsiate on Energy Balance: Critical Review and Meta-Analyses of Studies in Humans." *Chemical Senses* 37, no. 2 (2012): 103–21. doi:10.1093/chemse/bjr100.

53. Dalkara, Turgay and Kivilcim Kiliç. "How Does Fasting Trigger Migraine? A Hypothesis." *Current Pain and Headache Reports* 17, no. 10 (2013): 368. doi:10.1007/s11916-013-0368-1.

54. Kurosawa, Yuko, et al. "Creatine Supplementation Enhances Anaerobic ATP Synthesis During a Single 10 Sec Maximal Handgrip Exercise." *Molecular and Cellular Biochemistry* 244, nos. 1–2 (2003): 105–12; Pan, J.W. and K. Takahashi. "Cerebral Energetic Effects of Creatine Supplementation in Humans." *American Journal of Physiology. Regulatory, Integrative, and Comparative Physiology* 292, no. 4 (2007): R1745–50. doi:10.1152/ajpregu.00717.2006.

55. Futatsuki, Takahiro, et al. "Involvement of Orexin Neurons in Fasting- and Central Adenosine-Induced Hypothermia." *Scientific Reports* 8, no. 1 (2018): 2717. doi:10.1038/s41598-018-21252-w.

Chapter 5: Breaking Your Fast

1. Oarada, M., et al. "Refeeding with a High-Protein Diet After a 48 H Fast Causes Acute Hepatocellular Injury in Mice." *British Journal of Nutrition* 107, no. 10 (2012): 1435–1444. doi:10.1017/S0007114511004521.

2. Abdeen, S., et al. "Fasting-Induced Intestinal Damage is Mediated by Oxidative and Inflammatory Responses." *British Journal of Surgery* 96, no. 5 (2009): 552–9. doi:10.1002/bjs.6588.

3. Ottosson, M., et al. "The Effects of Cortisol on the Regulation of Lipoprotein Lipase Activity in Human Adipose Tissue." *The Journal of Clinical Endocrinology & Metabolism* 79, no. 3 (1994): 820–5. doi:10.1210/jcem.79.3.8077367.

4. McLaughlan, Eleanor and Julian H. Barth. "An Analysis of the Relationship Between Serum Cortisol and Serum Sodium in Routine Clinical Patients." *Practical Laboratory Medicine* 8 (2017): 30–33. doi:10.1016/j.plabm.2017.04.003.

5. Aguilera, G., et al. "Control of Aldosterone Secretion During Sodium Restriction: Adrenal Receptor Regulation and Increased Adrenal Sensitivity to Angiotensin II." *Proceedings of the National Academy of Sciences of the United States of America* 75, no. 2 (1978): 975–9. doi:10.1073/pnas.75.2.975.

6. Sartori, S.B., et al. "Magnesium Deficiency Induces Anxiety and HPA Axis Dysregulation: Modulation by Therapeutic Drug Treatment." *Neuropharmacology* 62, no. 1 (2012): 304–12. doi:10.1016/j.neuropharm.2011.07.027.

7. Martens, Mieke J.I., et al. "Effects of Single Macronutrients on Serum Cortisol Concentrations in Normal Weight Men." *Physiology & Behavior* 101, no. 5 (2010): 563–7. doi:10.1016/j.physbeh.2010.09.007.

8. Daley, C.A., et al. "A Review of Fatty Acid Profiles and Antioxidant Content in Grass-Fed and Grain-Fed Beef." *Nutrition Journal* 9, no. 10 (2010). doi:10.1186/1475-2891-9-10; Liu, Ying-Hua, et al. "Omega-3 Fatty Acid Intervention Suppresses Lipopolysaccharide-Induced Inflammation and Weight Loss in Mice." *Marine Drugs* 13, no. 2 (2015): 1026–36. doi:10.3390/md13021026.

9. Briet, Francoise, et al. "Effect of Malnutrition and Short-Term Refeeding on Peripheral Blood Mononuclear Cell Mitochondrial Complex I Activity in Humans." *The American Journal of Clinical Nutrition* 77, no. 5 (2003): 1304–1311. doi:10.1093/ajcn/77.5.1304.

10. Castro, Marta Araujo and Clotilde Vázquez Martínez. "The Refeeding Syndrome. Importance of Phosphorus." "El síndrome de realimentación. Importancia del fósforo." *Medicina Clinica* 150, no. 12 (2018): 472–478. doi:10.1016/j.medcli.2017.12.008; Stanga, Z., et al. "Nutrition in Clinical Practice—The Refeeding Syndrome: Illustrative Cases and Guidelines for Prevention and Treatment." *European Journal of Clinical Nutrition* 62 (2008): 687–694. doi:10.1038/sj.ejcn.1602854.

11. Lyte, Joshua M., et al. "Postprandial Serum Endotoxin in Healthy Humans Is Modulated by Dietary Fat in a Randomized, Controlled, Crossover Study." *Lipids in Health and Disease* 15, no. 1 (2016): 186. doi:10.1186/s12944-016-0357-6.

12. Ahrén, B., et al. "Acylation Stimulating Protein Stimulates Insulin Secretion." *International Journal of Obesity and Related Metabolic Disorders* 27, no. 9 (2003): 1037–43. doi:10.1038/sj.ijo.0802369; Cianflone, Katherine, et al. "Critical Review of Acylation-Stimulating Protein Physiology in Humans and Rodents." *Biochimica et Biophysica Acta (BBA)—Biomembranes* 1609, no. 2 (2003): 127–143. doi:10.1016/S0005-2736(02)00686-7.

13. Huppertz, T., et al. "3—The Caseins: Structure, Stability, and Functionality." in *Proteins in Food Processing* (2nd ed.), Woodhead Publishing Series in Food Science, Technology, and Nutrition. Cambridge, UK: Woodhead Publishing, 2018.

14. Brooke-Taylor, Simon, et al. "Systematic Review of the Gastrointestinal Effects of A1 Compared with A2 β-Casein." *Advances in Nutrition* 8, no. 5 (2017): 739–748. doi:10.3945/an.116.013953; Haq, Ul, et al. "Comparative Evaluation of Cow β-casein Variants (A1/A2) Consumption on Th2-Mediated Inflammatory Response in Mouse Gut." *European Journal of Nutrition* 53, no. 4 (2014): 1039–49. doi:10.1007/s00394-013-0606-7; Jianqin, Sun, et al. "Effects of Milk Containing Only A2 Beta Casein versus Milk Containing Both A1 and A2 Beta Casein Proteins on Gastrointestinal Physiology, Symptoms of Discomfort, and Cognitive Behavior of People with Self-Reported Intolerance to Traditional Cow's Milk." *Nutrition Journal* 15 (2016): 35. doi:10.1186/s12937-016-0147-z.

15. Ho, S., et al. "Comparative Effects of A1 versus A2 Beta-Casein on Gastrointestinal Measures: A Blinded Randomised Crossover Pilot Study." *European Journal of Clinical Nutrition* 68, no. 9 (2014): 994–1000. doi:10.1038/ejcn.2014.127; Guantario, Barbara, et al. "A Comprehensive Evaluation of the Impact of Bovine Milk Containing Different Beta-Casein Profiles on Gut

Health of Aging Mice." *Nutrients* 12, no. 7 (2020): 2147. doi:10.3390/nu12072147.

16. Vasconcelos, Ilka M. and José Tadeu A. Oliveira. "Antinutritional Properties of Plant Lectins." *Toxicon* 44, no. 4 (2004): 385–403. doi:10.1016/j.toxicon.2004.05.005.

17. Bohn, T., et al. "Fractional Magnesium Absorption Is Significantly Lower in Human Subjects from a Meal Served with an Oxalate-Rich Vegetable, Spinach, as Compared with a Meal Served with Kale, a Vegetable with a Low Oxalate Content." *British Journal of Nutrition* 91, no. 4 (2004): 601–606. doi:10.1079/BJN20031081.

18. Schlemmer, Ulrich, et al. "Phytate in Foods and Significance for Humans: Food Sources, Intake, Processing, Bioavailability, Protective Role, and Analysis." *Molecular Nutrition & Food Research* 53, no. 2 (2009): S330–75. doi:10.1002/mnfr.200900099.

19. Lammers, Karen M., et al. "Gliadin Induces an Increase in Intestinal Permeability and Zonulin Release by Binding to the Chemokine Receptor CXCR3." *Gastroenterology* 135, no. 1 (2008): 194–204.e3. doi:10.1053/j.gastro.2008.03.023; Vojdani, Aristo and Igal Tarash. "Cross-Reaction Between Gliadin and Different Food and Tissue Antigens." *Food and Nutrition Sciences* 4, no. 1 (2013): 20–32. doi:10.4236/fns.2013.41005; Lerner, Aaron, et al. "Gut-Thyroid Axis and Celiac Disease." *Endocrine Connections* 6, no. 4 (2017): R52–R58. doi:10.1530/EC-17-0021; Naiyer, Afzal, et al. "Tissue Transglutaminase Antibodies in Individuals with Celiac Disease Bind to Thyroid Follicles and Extracellular Matrix and May Contribute to Thyroid Dysfunction." *Thyroid* 18, no. 11 (2008): 1171–8. doi:10.1089/thy.2008.0110.

20. Vojdani, Aristo. "Lectins, Agglutinins, and Their Roles in Autoimmune Reactivities." *Alternative Therapies in Health and Medicine* 21, no. 1 (2015): 46–51. PMID:25599185.

21. Abdeen, S., et al. "Fasting-Induced Intestinal Damage Is Mediated by Oxidative and Inflammatory Responses." *British Journal of Surgery* 96, no. 5 (2009): 552–9. doi:10.1002/bjs.6588.

22. Rao, Radha Krishna and Geetha Samak. "Role of Glutamine in Protection of Intestinal Epithelial Tight Junctions." *Journal of Epithelial Biology & Pharmacology* 5, Suppl 1–M7 (2012): 47–54. doi:10.2174/1875044301205010047.

23. Smith, Gordon I., et al. "Dietary Omega-3 Fatty Acid Supplementation Increases the Rate of Muscle Protein Synthesis in Older Adults: A Randomized Controlled Trial." *The American Journal of Clinical Nutrition* 93, no. 2 (2011): 402–12. doi:10.3945/ajcn.110.005611; Traba, Javier, et al. "Fasting and Refeeding Differentially Regulate NLRP3 Inflammasome Activation in Human Subjects." *The Journal of Clinical Investigation* 125, no. 12 (2015): 4592–4600. doi:10.1172/JCI83260.

24. Brighenti, F., et al. "Effect of Neutralized and Native Vinegar on Blood Glucose and Acetate Responses to a Mixed Meal in Healthy Subjects." *European Journal of Clinical Nutrition* 49, no. 4 (1995): 242–7. PMID:7796781; Bjarnsholt, Thomas, et al. "Antibiofilm Properties of Acetic Acid." *Advances in Wound Care* 4, no. 7 (2015): 363–372. doi:10.1089/wound.2014.0554.

25. Zbigniew, Szybinski. "Role of Iodine in Metabolism." *Recent Patents on Endocrine, Metabolic & Immune Drug Discovery* 10, no. 2 (2017): 123–126. doi:10.2174/1872214811666170119110618.

26. Fuehrlein, Brian S., et al. "Differential Metabolic Effects of Saturated *versus* Polyunsaturated Fats in Ketogenic Diets." *The Journal of Clinical Endocrinology & Metabolism* 89: 4 (2004): 1641–1645. doi:org/10.1210/jc.2003-031796.

27. Carrillo, C., et al. "Role of Oleic Acid in Immune System; Mechanism of Action; A Review." *Nutricion Hospitalaria* 27, no. 4 (2012): 978–90. doi:10.3305/nh.2012.27.4.5783; Basu, Arpita, et al. "Dietary Factors that Promote or Retard Inflammation." *Arteriosclerosis, Thrombosis, and Vascular Biology* 26, no. 5 (2006): 995–1001. doi:10.1161/01.ATV.0000214295.86079.d1; Kondo, Tomoo, et al. "Acetic Acid Upregulates the Expression of Genes for Fatty Acid Oxidation Enzymes in Liver to Suppress Body Fat Accumulation." *Journal of Agriculture and Food Chemistry* 57, no. 13 (2009): 5982–5986. doi:10.1021/jf900470c.

28. Lee, W., et al. "Anti-inflammatory Effects of Olean-olic Acid on LPS-Induced Inflammation *In Vitro* and *In Vivo*." *Inflammation* 36, (2013): 94–102. doi:10.1007/s10753-012-9523-9.

29. Lyte, Joshua M., et al. "Postprandial Serum Endo-toxin in Healthy Humans Is Modulated by Dietary Fat in a Randomized, Controlled, Crossover Study." *Lipids in Health and Disease* 15, no. 1 (2016): 186. doi:10.1186/s12944-016-0357-6.

30. Michnovicz, J.J. and H.L. Bradlow. "Altered Estrogen Metabolism and Excretion in Humans Following Consumption of Indole-3-Carbinol." *Nutrition and Cancer* 16, no. 1 (1991): 59–66. doi:10.1080/01635589109514141.

31. Knudsen, Bach, et al. "Impact of Diet-Modulated Butyrate Production on Intestinal Barrier Function and Inflammation." *Nutrients* 10, no. 10 (2018): 1499. doi:10.3390/nu10101499; Li, Z., et al. "Butyrate Reduces Appetite and Activates Brown Adipose Tissue via the Gut-Brain Neural Circuit." *Gut* 67 (2018): 1269–1279. doi:10.1136/gutjnl-2017-314050.

32. Maciejak, P., et al. "Is the Interaction Between Fatty Acids and Tryptophan Responsible for the Efficacy of a Ketogenic Diet in Epilepsy? The New Hypothesis of Action." *Neuroscience* 313 (2016): 130–48. doi:10.1016/j.neuroscience.2015.11.029.

33. Yoon, Mee-Sup. "The Role of Mammalian Target of Rapamycin (mTOR) in Insulin Signaling." *Nutrients* 9, no. 11 (2017): 1176. doi:10.3390/nu9111176.

34. Solomon, S.M. and D.F. Kirby. "The Refeeding Syndrome: A Review." *Journal of Parenteral and Enteral Nutrition* 14, no. 1 (1990): 90–97. doi:10.1177/014860719001400190.

35. DePhillipo, Nicholas N., et al. "Efficacy of Vitamin C Supplementation on Collagen Synthesis and Oxidative Stress After Musculoskeletal Injuries: A Systematic Review." *Orthopaedic Journal of Sports Medicine* 6, no. 10 (2018). doi:10.1177/2325967118804544.

36. Smith, Gordon I., et al. "Dietary Omega-3 Fatty Acid Supplementation Increases the Rate of Muscle Protein Synthesis in Older Adults: A Randomized Con-trolled Trial." *The American Journal of Clinical Nutrition* 93, no. 2 (2011): 402–12. doi:10.3945/ajcn.110.005611; Traba, Javier, et al. "Fasting and Refeeding Differen-tially Regulate NLRP3 Inflammasome Activation in Human Subjects." *The Journal of Clinical Investigation* 125, no. 12 (2015): 4592–4600. doi:10.1172/JCI83260.

37. Brighenti, F., et al. "Effect of Neutralized and Native Vinegar on Blood Glucose and Acetate Responses to a Mixed Meal in Healthy Subjects." *European Journal of Clinical Nutrition* 49, no. 4 (1995): 242–7. PMID:7796781; Bjarnsholt, Thomas, et al. "Antibiofilm Properties of Acetic Acid." *Advances in Wound Care* 4, no. 7 (2015): 363–372. doi:10.1089/wound.2014.0554.

38. Rao, Radha Krishna and Geetha Samak. "Role of Glutamine in Protection of Intestinal Epithelial Tight Junctions." *Journal of Epithelial Biology & Pharmacology* 5, Suppl 1–M7 (2012): 47–54. doi:10.2174/1875044301205010047.

39. Knudsen, Bach, et al. "Impact of Diet-Modulated Butyrate Production on Intestinal Barrier Function and Inflammation." *Nutrients* 10, no. 10 (2018): 1499. doi:10.3390/nu10101499; Li, Z., et al. "Butyrate Reduces Appetite and Activates Brown Adipose Tissue via the Gut-Brain Neural Circuit." *Gut* 67 (2018): 1269–1279. doi:10.1136/gutjnl-2017-314050.

40. Maciejak, P., et al. "Is the Interaction Between Fatty Acids and Tryptophan Responsible for the Efficacy of a Ketogenic Diet in Epilepsy? The New Hypothesis of Action." *Neuroscience* 313 (2016): 130–48. doi:10.1016/j.neuroscience.2015.11.029.

41. Sanders, T.A. and S. Reddy. "The Influence of a Vegetarian Diet on the Fatty Acid Composition of Human Milk and the Essential Fatty Acid Status of the Infant." *The Journal of Pediatrics* 120, no. 4 Pt 2 (1992): S71–7. doi:10.1016/s0022-3476(05)81239-9.

42. Smith, Gordon I., et al. "Dietary Omega-3 Fatty Acid Supplementation Increases the Rate of Muscle Protein Synthesis in Older Adults: A Randomized Con-trolled Trial." *The American Journal of Clinical Nutrition* 93, no. 2 (2011): 402–12. doi:10.3945/ajcn.110.005611; Traba, Javier, et al. "Fasting and Refeeding Differen-tially Regulate NLRP3 Inflammasome Activation in Human Subjects." *The Journal of Clinical Investigation* 125, no. 12 (2015): 4592–4600. doi:10.1172/JCI83260.

43. Mindikoglu, Ayse L., et al. "Intermittent Fasting from Dawn to Sunset for 30 Consecutive Days Is Associated with Anticancer Proteomic Signature and Upregulates Key Regulatory Proteins of Glucose and Lipid Metabolism, Circadian Clock, DNA Repair, Cytoskeleton Remodeling, Immune System, and Cognitive Function in Healthy Subjects." *Journal of Proteomics* 217 (2020): 103645. doi:10.1016/j.jprot.2020.103645.

44. Nakamura, Takahisa, et al. "Double-Stranded RNA-Dependent Protein Kinase Links Pathogen Sensing with Stress and Metabolic Homeostasis." *Cell* 140 (2010): 338–348. doi:10.1016/j.cell.2010.01.001.

45. Leidy, Heather J., et al. "The Role of Protein in Weight Loss and Maintenance." *The American Journal of Clinical Nutrition* 101, no. 6 (2015): 1320S–1329S. doi:10.3945/ajcn.114.084038.

46. Gosby, Alison K., et al. "Testing Protein Leverage in Lean Humans: A Randomised Controlled Experimental Study." *PLOS One* 6, no. 10 (2011): e25929. doi:10.1371/journal.pone.0025929.

47. Cassady, Bridget A., et al. "Mastication of Almonds: Effects of Lipid Bioaccessibility, Appetite, and Hormone Response." *The American Journal of Clinical Nutrition* 89, no. 3 (2009): 794–800. doi:10.3945/ajcn.2008.26669; Li, Jie, et al. "Improvement in Chewing Activity Reduces Energy Intake in One Meal and Modulates Plasma Gut Hormone Concentrations in Obese and Lean Young Chinese Men." *The American Journal of Clinical Nutrition* 94, no. 3 (2011): 709–16. doi:10.3945/ajcn.111.015164.

48. Halmos, Emma P., et al. "A Diet Low in FODMAPs Reduces Symptoms of Irritable Bowel Syndrome." *Gastroenterology* 146, no. 1 (2014): 67–75.e5. doi:10.1053/j.gastro.2013.09.046.

49. Oben, Julius, et al. "An Open Label Study to Determine the Effects of an Oral Proteolytic Enzyme System on Whey Protein Concentrate Metabolism in Healthy Males." *Journal of the International Society of Sports Nutrition* 5, no. 10 (2008). doi:10.1186/1550-2783-5-10.

50. Folkers, K., et al. "Lovastatin Decreases Coenzyme Q Levels in Humans." *Proceedings of the National Academy of Sciences of the United States of America* 87, no. 22 (1990): 8931–4. doi:10.1073/pnas.87.22.8931.

51. Hori, Juliana I., et al. "The Inhibition of Inflammasome by Brazilian Propolis (EPP-AF)." *Evidence-Based Complementary and Alternative Medicine* 2013 (2013). doi:10.1155/2013/418508.

52. Pasupuleti, Visweswara Rao, et al. "Honey, Propolis, and Royal Jelly: A Comprehensive Review of Their Biological Actions and Health Benefits." *Oxidative Medicine and Cellular Longevity* 2017 (2017). doi:10.1155/2017/1259510.

Chapter 6: Your Eating Window

1. Rizzo, Nico, et al. "Nutrient Profiles of Vegetarian and Nonvegetarian Dietary Patterns." *Journal of the Academy of Nutrition and Dietetics* 113, no. 12 (2013): 1610–9. doi:10.1016/j.jand.2013.06.349.

2. Estruch, Ramón, et al. "Primary Prevention of Cardiovascular Disease with a Mediterranean Diet Supplemented with Extra-Virgin Olive Oil or Nuts." *The New England Journal of Medicine* 378, no. 25 (2018): e34. doi:10.1056/NEJMoa1800389; Fitó, M., et al. "Effect of a Traditional Mediterranean Diet on Lipoprotein Oxidation: A Randomized Controlled Trial." *Archives of Internal Medicine* 167, no. 11 (2007): 1195–1203. doi:10.1001/archinte.167.11.1195; Shai, I., et al. "Weight Loss with a Low-Carbohydrate, Mediterranean, or Low-Fat Diet." *The New England Journal of Medicine* 359, no. 3 (2008): 229–241. doi:10.1056/nejmoa0708681.

3. Paniagua, J.A., et al. "Monounsaturated Fat–Rich Diet Prevents Central Body Fat Distribution and Decreases Postprandial Adiponectin Expression Induced by a Carbohydrate-Rich Diet in Insulin-Resistant Subjects." *Diabetes Care* 30, no. 7 (2007): 1717–1723. doi:10.2337/dc06-2220.

4. Mindikoglu, Ayse L., et al. "Intermittent Fasting from Dawn to Sunset for 30 Consecutive Days Is Associated with Anticancer Proteomic Signature and Upregulates Key Regulatory Proteins of Glucose and Lipid Metabolism, Circadian Clock, DNA Repair, Cytoskeleton Remodeling, Immune System, and Cognitive Function in Healthy Subjects." *Journal of Proteomics* 217 (2020). doi:10.1016/j.jprot.2020.103645.

5. Dimitrov, Dimiter. "Effect of Omega-3 Fatty Acids on Plasma Adiponectin Levels in Metabolic Syndrome Subjects." *International Journal of Obesity* 31 (2007): S34–S34.

6. Sabarwal, Akash, et al. "Hazardous Effects of Chemical Pesticides on Human Health–Cancer and Other Associated Disorders." *Environmental Toxicology and Pharmacology* 63 (2018): 103–114. doi:10.1016/j.etap.2018.08.018; Yan, D., et al. "Pesticide Exposure and Risk of Alzheimer's Disease: A Systematic Review and Meta-Analysis." *Scientific Reports* 6, no. 32222 (2016). doi:10.1038/srep32222.

7. Malekinejad, Hassan and Aysa Rezabakhsh. "Hormones in Dairy Foods and Their Impact on Public Health—A Narrative Review Article." *Iranian Journal of Public Health* 44, no. 6 (2015): 742–58.

8. Qi, K., et al. "Rearing Pattern Alters Porcine Myofiber Type, Fat Deposition, Associated Microbial Communities, and Functional Capacity." *BMC Microbiology* 19 (2019): 181. doi:10.1186/s12866-019-1556-x.

9. EDF Seafood Selector. Mercury in Seafood. https://seafood.edf.org/mercury-seafood.

10. EDF Seafood Selector. Common Questions About Contaminants in Seafood. https://seafood.edf.org /common-questions-about-contaminants-seafood.

11. Oomen, C.M., et al. "Association Between Trans Fatty Acid Intake and 10-Year Risk of Coronary Heart Disease in the Zutphen Elderly Study: A Prospective Population-Based Study." *Lancet* 357, no. 9258 (2001): 746–51. doi:10.1016/s0140-6736(00)04166-0; Oh, Kyungwon, et al. "Dietary Fat Intake and Risk of Coronary Heart Disease in Women: 20 Years of Follow-Up of the Nurses' Health Study." *American Journal of Epidemiology* 161, no. 7 (2005): 672–9. doi:10.1093/aje /kwi085; Kavanagh, Kylie, et al. "Trans Fat Diet Induces Abdominal Obesity and Changes in Insulin Sensitivity in Monkeys." *Obesity* 15, no. 7 (2007): 1675–84. doi:10.1038/oby.2007.200.

12. Tey, S.L., et al. "Effects of Aspartame-, Monk Fruit-, Stevia- and Sucrose-Sweetened Beverages on Postprandial Glucose, Insulin, and Energy Intake." *International Journal of Obesity* 41, no. 3 (2017): 450–457. doi:10.1038/ijo.2016.225; Goyal, S.K., et al. "Stevia (*Stevia rebaudiana*): A Bio-Sweetener: A Review." *International Journal of Food Sciences and Nutrition* 61, no. 1 (2010): 1–10. doi:10.3109/09637480903193049; Xu, Q., et al. "Antioxidant Effect of Mogrosides Against Oxidative Stress Induced by Palmitic Acid in Mouse Insulinoma NIT-1 Cells." *Brazilian Journal of Medical and Biological Research = Revista brasileira de pesquisas medicas e biologicas* 46, no. 11 (2013): 949–955. doi:10.1590/1414-431X20133163.

13. Brooke-Taylor, Simon, et al. "Systematic Review of the Gastrointestinal Effects of A1 Compared with A2 β-Casein." *Advances in Nutrition* 8, no. 5 (2017): 739–748. doi:10.3945/an.116.013953; Haq, Ul, et al. "Comparative Evaluation of Cow β-casein Variants (A1/A2) Consumption on Th2-Mediated Inflammatory Response in Mouse Gut." European Journal of Nutrition 53, no. 4 (2014): 1039–49. doi:10.1007 /s00394-013-0606-7; Jianqin, Sun, et al. "Effects of Milk Containing Only A2 Beta Casein versus Milk Containing Both A1 and A2 Beta Casein Proteins on Gastrointestinal Physiology, Symptoms of Discomfort, and Cognitive Behavior of People with Self-Reported Intolerance to Traditional Cow's Milk." *Nutrition Journal* 15 (2016): 35. doi:10.1186/s12937-016-0147-z.

14. Malekinejad, Hassan and Aysa Rezabakhsh. "Hormones in Dairy Foods and Their Impact on Public Health—A Narrative Review Article." *Iranian Journal of Public Health* 44, no. 6 (2015): 742–58.

15. Jianqin, Sun, et al. "Effects of Milk Containing Only A2 Beta Casein versus Milk Containing Both A1 and A2 Beta Casein Proteins on Gastrointestinal Physiology, Symptoms of Discomfort, and Cognitive Behavior of People with Self-Reported Intolerance to Traditional Cow's Milk." *Nutrition Journal* 15 (2016): 35. doi:10.1186 /s12937-016-0147-z.

16. Lenoir, Magalie, et al. "Intense Sweetness Surpasses Cocaine Reward." *PLOS One* 2, no. 8 (2007): e698. doi:10.1371/journal.pone.0000698; Avena, Nicole M., et al. "Evidence for Sugar Addiction: Behavioral and Neurochemical Effects of Intermittent, Excessive Sugar Intake." *Neuroscience and Biobehavioral Reviews* 32, no. 1 (2008): 20–39. doi:10.1016 /j.neubiorev.2007.04.019.

17. DiNicolantonio, James J. and James H. OKeefe. "Added Sugars Drive Coronary Heart Disease via Insulin Resistance and Hyperinsulinaemia: A New Paradigm." *Open Heart* 4, no. 2 (2017): e000729. doi:10.1136/openhrt-2017-000729; Malik, Vasanti S., et al. "Sugar-Sweetened Beverages, Obesity, Type 2 Diabetes Mellitus, and Cardiovascular Disease Risk." *Circulation* 121, no. 11 (2010): 1356–64. doi:10.1161/CIRCULATIONAHA.109.876185.

18. University of California San Francisco, Sugar Science, The Unsweetened Truth. "Hidden in Plain Sight." https://sugarscience.ucsf.edu/hidden-in-plain-sight/#.YGYIIS1hOUQ.

19. Yang, Qing. "Gain Weight by 'Going Diet?' Artificial Sweeteners and the Neurobiology of Sugar Cravings: Neuroscience 2010." *The Yale Journal of Biology and Medicine* 83, no. 2 (2010): 101–8. PMID:20589192.

20. Lennon, E.J. and W.F. Piering. "A Comparison of the Effects of Glucose Ingestion and NH4Cl Acidosis on Urinary Calcium and Magnesium Excretion in Man." *The Journal of Clinical Investigation* 49, no. 7 (1970): 1458–65. doi:10.1172/JCI106363; Chen, Ling, et al. "Hyperglycemia Inhibits the Uptake of Dehydroascorbate in Tubular Epithelial Cell." *American Journal of Nephrology* 25, no. 5 (2005): 459–65. doi:10.1159/000087853; Brenza, Holly L., et al. "Parathyroid Hormone Activation of the 25-hydroxyvitamin D3-1α-hydroxylase Gene Promoter." *Proceedings of the National Academy of Sciences* 95, no. 4 (1998): 1387–1391. doi:10.1073/pnas.95.4.1387.

21. Innes, Jacqueline K., and Philip C. Calder. "Omega-6 Fatty Acids and Inflammation." *Prostaglandins, Leukotrienes, and Essential Fatty Acids* 132 (2018): 41–48. doi:10.1016/j.plefa.2018.03.004.

22. Balakireva, Anastasia V. and Andrey A. Zamyatnin. "Properties of Gluten Intolerance: Gluten Structure, Evolution, Pathogenicity, and Detoxification Capabilities." *Nutrients* 8, no. 10 (2016): 644. doi:10.3390/nu8100644; de Punder, Karin and Leo Pruimboom. "The Dietary Intake of Wheat and Other Cereal Grains and Their Role in Inflammation." *Nutrients* 5, no. 3 (2013): 771–87. doi:10.3390/nu5030771.

23. de Punder, Karin and Leo Pruimboom. "The Dietary Intake of Wheat and Other Cereal Grains and Their Role in Inflammation." *Nutrients* 5, no. 3 (2013): 771–87. doi:10.3390/nu5030771.

24. Marklund, Matti, et al. "Biomarkers of Dietary Omega-6 Fatty Acids and Incident Cardiovascular Disease and Mortality." *Circulation* 139, no. 21 (2019): 2422–2436. doi:10.1161/CIRCULATIONAHA.118.038908

25. Garrido-Maraver, Juan, et al. "Coenzyme q10 Therapy." *Molecular Syndromology* 5, nos. 3–4 (2014): 187–97. doi:10.1159/000360101.

26. Naghii, Mohammad Reza, et al. "Comparative Effects of Daily and Weekly Boron Supplementation on Plasma Steroid Hormones and Proinflammatory Cytokines." *Journal of Trace Elements in Medicine and Biology: Organ of the Society for Minerals and Trace Elements (GMS)* 25, no. 1 (2011): 54–8. doi:10.1016/j.jtemb.2010.10.001; Ferrando, A.A. and N.R. Green. "The Effect of Boron Supplementation on Lean Body Mass, Plasma Testosterone Levels, and Strength in Male Bodybuilders." *International Journal of Sport Nutrition* 3, no. 2 (1993): 140–9. doi:10.1123/ijsn.3.2.140.

27. National Institutes of Health. "Boron: Fact Sheet for Health Professionals." https://ods.od.nih.gov/factsheets/Boron-HealthProfessional/.

28. Pilchova, Ivana, et al. "The Involvement of Mg2+ in Regulation of Cellular and Mitochondrial Functions." *Oxidative Medicine and Cellular Longevity* (2017). doi:10.1155/2017/6797460.

29. Kostov, Krasimir. "Effects of Magnesium Deficiency on Mechanisms of Insulin Resistance in Type 2 Diabetes: Focusing on the Processes of Insulin Secretion and Signaling." *International Journal of Molecular Sciences* 20, no. 6 (2019): 1351. doi:10.3390/ijms20061351.

30. Smith, Gordon I., et al. "Dietary Omega-3 Fatty Acid Supplementation Increases the Rate of Muscle Protein Synthesis in Older Adults: A Randomized Controlled Trial." *The American Journal of Clinical Nutrition* 93, no. 2 (2011): 402–12. doi:10.3945/ajcn.110.005611; Traba, Javier, et al. "Fasting and Refeeding Differentially Regulate NLRP3 Inflammasome Activation in Human Subjects." *The Journal of Clinical Investigation*

125, no. 12 (2015): 4592–4600. doi:10.1172/JCI83260; Rathod, R., et al. "Novel Insights into the Effect of Vitamin B_{12} and Omega-3 Fatty Acids on Brain Function." *Journal of Biomedical Science* 23 (2016): 17. doi:10.1186/s12929-016-0241-8.

31. Sanders, T.A. and S. Reddy. "The Influence of a Vegetarian Diet on the Fatty Acid Composition of Human Milk and the Essential Fatty Acid Status of the Infant." *The Journal of Pediatrics* 120, no. 4 Pt 2 (1992): S71–7. doi:10.1016/s0022-3476(05)81239-9.

32. Rathod, R., et al. "Novel Insights into the Effect of Vitamin B_{12} and Omega-3 Fatty Acids on Brain Function." *Journal of Biomedical Science* 23 (2016): 17. doi:10.1186/s12929-016-0241-8.

33. Rafiq, Rachida, et al. "Associations of Different Body Fat Deposits with Serum 25-Hydroxyvitamin D Concentrations." *Clinical* 38, no. 6 (2019): 2851–2857. doi:10.1016/j.clnu.2018.12.018.

34. Remelli, Francesca, et al. "Vitamin D Deficiency and Sarcopenia in Older Persons." *Nutrients* 11, no. 12 (2019): 2861. doi:10.3390/nu11122861.

35. Calton, E.K., et al. "Vitamin D Status and Insulin Sensitivity Are Novel Predictors of Resting Metabolic Rate: A Cross-Sectional Analysis in Australian Adults." *European Journal of Nutrition* 55 (2016): 2075–2080. doi:10.1007/s00394-015-1021-z.

36. Daxenberger, A., et al. "Increased Milk Levels of Insulinlike Growth Factor 1 (IGF-1) for the Identification of Bovine Somatotropin (bST) Treated Cows." *The Analyst* 123, no. 12 (1998): 2429–35. doi:10.1039/a804923h.

37. Malekinejad, Hassan and Aysa Rezabakhsh. "Hormones in Dairy Foods and Their Impact on Public Health—A Narrative Review Article." *Iranian Journal of Public Health* 44, no. 6 (2015): 742–58.

38. Fothergill, E., et al. "Persistent Metabolic Adaptation 6 Years After *The Biggest Loser* Competition." *Obesity* 24 (2016): 1612–1619. doi:10.1002/oby.21538.

39. Mulder, H., et al. "Melatonin Receptors in Pancreatic Islets: Good Morning to a Novel Type 2 Diabetes Gene." *Diabetologia* 52, no.7 (2009): 1240–9. doi:10.1007/s00125-009-1359-y.

40. Kahleova, Hana, et al. "Eating Two Larger Meals a Day (Breakfast and Lunch) Is More Effective than Six Smaller Meals in a Reduced-Energy Regimen for Patients with Type 2 Diabetes: A Randomised Crossover Study." *Diabetologia* 57, no. 8 (2014): 1552–60. doi:10.1007/s00125-014-3253-5.

Chapter 8: Supercharge Fat Burning

1. Bracken, R., et al. "Plasma Catecholamine and Nephrine Responses to Brief Intermittent Maximal Intensity Exercise." *Amino Acids* 36 (2008): 209–217. doi:10.1007/s00726-008-0049-2.

2. Senf, Sarah M. "Skeletal Muscle Heat Shock Protein 70: Diverse Functions and Therapeutic Potential for Wasting Disorders." *Frontiers in Physiology* 4 (2013): 330. doi:10.3389/fphys.2013.00330; Laukkanen, Jari A., et al. "Cardiovascular and Other Health Benefits of Sauna Bathing: A Review of the Evidence." *Mayo Clinic Proceedings* 93, no. 8 (2018): 1111–1121. doi:10.1016/j.mayocp.2018.04.008.

3. Pilch, Wanda, et al. "Changes in the Lipid Profile of Blood Serum in Women Taking Sauna Baths of Various Duration." *International Journal of Occupational Medicine and Environmental Health* 23, no. 2 (2010): 167–74. doi:10.2478/v10001-010-0020-9.

4. Cahill Jr., George F. "Fuel Metabolism in Starvation." I>Annual Review of Nutrition 26, no. 1 (2006): 1–22. doi:10.1146/annurev.nutr.26.061505.111258.

5. Tinsley, Grant M. and Paul M. La Bounty. "Effects of Intermittent Fasting on Body Composition and Clinical Health Markers in Humans." *Nutrition Reviews* 73, no. 10 (2015): 661–674. doi:10.1093/nutrit/nuv041.

6. Gonzalez, Javier T., et al. "Breakfast and Exercise Contingently Affect Postprandial Metabolism and Energy Balance in Physically Active Males." *British Journal of Nutrition* 110, no. 4 (2013): 721–32. doi:10.1017/S0007114512005582.

7. Tinsley, Grant M. and Paul M. La Bounty. "Effects of Intermittent Fasting on Body Composition and Clinical Health Markers in Humans." *Nutrition Reviews* 73, no. 10 (2015): 661–674. doi:10.1093/nutrit/nuv041.

8. Stekovic, Steven, et al. "Alternate-Day Fasting Improves Physiological and Molecular Markers of Aging in Healthy, Non-Obese Humans." *Cell Metabolism* 30, no. 3 (2019): 462–476. doi:10.1016/j.cmet.2019.07.016.

9. Dyson, P.A., et al. "A Low-Carbohydrate Diet Is More Effective in Reducing Body Weight than Healthy Eating in Both Diabetic and Non-Diabetic Subjects." *Diabetic Medicine: A Journal of the British Diabetic Association* 24, no. 12 (2007): 1430–5. doi:10.1111/j.1464-5491.2007.02290.x.

10. Choi, Inho, et al. "The New Era of the Lymphatic System: No Longer Secondary to the Blood Vascular System." *Cold Spring Harbor Perspectives in Medicine* 2, no. 4 (2012): a006445. doi:10.1101/cshperspect.a006445; Breslin, Jerome, et al. "Lymphatic Vessel Network Structure and Physiology." *Comprehensive Physiology* 9, no. 1 (2018): 207–299. doi:10.1002/cphy.c180015.

11. Lane, Kirstin, et al. "Lymphoscintigraphy to Evaluate the Effect of High versus Low Intensity Upper Body Dynamic Exercise on Lymphatic Function in Healthy Females." *Lymphatic Research and Biology* 4, no. 3 (2006): 159–65. doi:10.1089/lrb.2006.4.159.

12. Lane, Kirstin, et al. "Exercise and the Lymphatic System: Implications for Breast-Cancer Survivors." *Sports Medicine* (Auckland, NZ) 35, no. 6 (2005): 461–71. doi:10.2165/00007256-200535060-00001.

13. Hase, Adrian, et al. "Behavioral and Cognitive Effects of Tyrosine Intake in Healthy Human Adults." *Pharmacology, Biochemistry, and Behavior* 133 (2015): 1–6. doi:10.1016/j.pbb.2015.03.008; Steenbergen, Laura, et al. "Tyrosine Promotes Cognitive Flexibility: Evidence from Proactive vs. Reactive Control During Task Switching Performance." *Neuropsychologia* 69 (2015): 50–5. doi:10.1016/j.neuropsychologia.2015.01.022

14. Hase, Adrian, et al. "Behavioral and Cognitive Effects of Tyrosine Intake in Healthy Human Adults." *Pharmacology, Biochemistry, and Behavior* 133 (2015): 1–6. doi:10.1016/j.pbb.2015.03.008.

15. Kurosawa, Yuko, et al. "Creatine Supplementation Enhances Anaerobic ATP Synthesis During a Single 10 Sec Maximal Handgrip Exercise." *Molecular and Cellular Biochemistry* 244, nos. 1–2 (2003): 105–12. PMID:12701817.

16. Walker, Dillon K., et al. "Exercise, Amino Acids, and Aging in the Control of Human Muscle Protein Synthesis." *Medicine and Science in Sports and Exercise* 43, no. 12 (2011): 2249–58. doi:10.1249/MSS.0b013e318223b037.

Chapter 9: Crush Inflammation

1. Furman, D., et al. "Chronic Inflammation in the Etiology of Disease Across the Life Span." *Nature Medicine* 25 (2019): 1822–1832 (2019). doi:10.1038/s41591-019-0675-0.

2. Faris, Mo'ez Al-Islam E., et al. "Intermittent Fasting During Ramadan Attenuates Proinflammatory Cytokines and Immune Cells in Healthy Subjects." *Nutrition Research* 32, no. 12 (2012): 947–55. doi:10.1016/j.nutres.2012.06.021.

3. Youm, Y.H., et al. "The Ketone Metabolite β-Hydroxybutyrate Blocks NLRP3 Inflammasome–Mediated Inflammatory Disease." *Nature Medicine* 21 (2015): 263–269. doi:10.1038/nm.3804.

4. Fann, David Yang-Wei, et al. "Intermittent Fasting Attenuates Inflammasome Activity in Ischemic Stroke." *Experimental Neurology* 257 (2014): 114–9. doi:10.1016/j.expneurol.2014.04.017.

5. Calder, Philip C. "Omega-3 Polyunsaturated Fatty Acids and Inflammatory Processes: Nutrition or Pharmacology?" *British Journal of Clinical Pharmacology* 75, no. 3 (2013): 645–62. doi:10.1111/j.1365-2125.2012.04374.x.

6. Calder, Philip C. "Omega-3 Polyunsaturated Fatty Acids and Inflammatory Processes: Nutrition or Pharmacology?" *British Journal of Clinical Pharmacology* 75, no. 3 (2013): 645–62. doi:10.1111/j.1365-2125.2012.04374.x.

7. Bailey, Stephen J., et al. "Dietary Nitrate Supplementation Reduces the O2 Cost of Low-Intensity Exercise and Enhances Tolerance to High-Intensity Exercise in Humans." *Journal of Applied Physiology* 2107, no. 4 (2009): 1144–1155. doi:10.1152/japplphysiol.00722.2009.

8. Clifford, Tom, et al. "The Potential Benefits of Red Beetroot Supplementation in Health and Disease." *Nutrients* 7, no. 4 (2015): 2801–22. doi:10.3390/nu7042801.

9. Zhao, Guangfu, et al. "Betaine in Inflammation: Mechanistic Aspects and Applications." *Frontiers in Immunology* 9 (2018): 1070. doi:10.3389/fimmu.2018.01070.

10. Donnarumma, Giovanna, et al. "AV119, a Natural Sugar from Avocado Gratissima, Modulates the LPS-Induced Proinflammatory Response in Human Heratinocytes." *Inflammation* 34, no. 6 (2011): 568–75. doi:10.1007/s10753-010-9264-6.

11. Jirillo, Felicita and Thea Magrone. "Anti-Inflammatory and Anti-Allergic Properties of Donkey's and Goat's Milk." *Endocrine, Metabolic & Immune Disorders—Drug Targets* 14, no. 1 (2014): 27–37. doi:10.2174/1871530314666140121143747.

12. Reygaert, Wanda C. "An Update on the Health Benefits of Green Tea." *Beverages* 3, no. 1 (2017): 6. doi:10.3390/beverages3010006.

13. Parkinson, Lisa and Russell Keast. "Oleocanthal, a Phenolic Derived from Virgin Olive Oil: A Review of the Beneficial Effects on Inflammatory Disease." *International Journal of Molecular Sciences* 15, no. 7 (2014): 12323–34. doi:10.3390/ijms150712323.

14. Belcaro, Gianni, et al. "Efficacy and Safety of Meriva®, a Curcumin-Phosphatidylcholine Complex, During Extended Administration in Osteoarthritis Patients." *Alternative Medicine Review: A Journal of Clinical Therapeutic* 15, no. 4 (2010): 337–44. PMID:21194249.

15. Chandran, Binu and Ajay Goel. "A Randomized, Pilot Study to Assess the Efficacy and Safety of Curcumin in Patients with Active Rheumatoid Arthritis." *Phytotherapy Research: PTR* 26, no. 11 (2012): 1719–25. doi:10.1002/ptr.4639.

16. Zhaoping, Li, et al. "Hass Avocado Modulates Postprandial Vascular Reactivity and Postprandial Inflammatory Responses to a Hamburger Meal in Healthy Volunteers." *Food & Function* 4, no. 3 (2013): 384–91. doi:10.1039/c2fo30226h.

17. Altman, R.D. and K.C. Marcussen. "Effects of a Ginger Extract on Knee Pain in Patients with Osteoarthritis." *Arthritis and Rheumatism* 44, no. 11 (2001): 2531–8. doi:10.1002/1529-0131(200111)44:11<2531::aid-art433>3.0.co;2-j.

18. Ha, S.K., et al. "6-Shogaol, a Ginger Product, Modulates Neuroinflammation: A New Approach to Neuroprotection." *Neuropharmacology* 63, no. 2 (2012): 211–23. doi:10.1016/j.neuropharm.2012.03.016.

19. United States Environmental Protection Agency. "Summary of the Toxic Substances Control Act." EPA.gov/laws-regulations/summary-toxic-substances-control-act.

20. United States Environmental Protection Agency. "Report to Congress on Indoor Air Quality: Volume 2." 1989. EPA/400/1-89/001C. Washington, DC; United States Environmental Protection Agency. "The Total Exposure Assessment Methodology (TEAM) Study: Summary and Analysis." 1987. EPA/600/6-87/002a. Washington, DC; United States Environmental Protection Agency. "Indoor Air Quality." EPA.gov/report-environment/indoor-air-quality.

21. Environmental Working Group. "EWG's Tap Water Database—2019 Update." EWG.org/tapwater/.

22. Dean, L. "Methylenetetrahydrofolate Reductase Deficiency." In Pratt, V.M., S.A. Scott, M. Pirmohamed, et al., eds. *Medical Genetics Summaries* [Internet] (March 8, 2012 [Updated October 27, 2016]). Bethesda, MD: National Center for Biotechnology Information (US). Available from ncbi.nlm.nih.gov/books/NBK66131/.

23. Sangouni, A., et al. "Effect of Garlic Powder Supplementation on Hepatic Steatosis, Liver Enzymes, and Lipid Profile in Patients with Non-Alcoholic Fatty Liver Disease: A Double-Blind Randomised Controlled Clinical Trial." *British Journal of Nutrition* 124, no. 4 (2020): 450–456. doi:10.1017/S0007114520001403.

24. Ried, Karin, et al. "Effect of Garlic on Serum Lipids: An Updated Meta-Analysis." *Nutrition Reviews* 71, no. 5 (2013): 282–99. doi:10.1111/nure.12012.

25. Bennett, Jeanette M., et al. "Inflammation and Reactivation of Latent Herpes Viruses in Older Adults." *Brain, Behavior, and Immunity* 26, no. 5 (2012): 739–46. doi:10.1016/j.bbi.2011.11.007.

26. Esch, P.M., et al. "Postoperative Schwellungsreduktion. Objektive Schwellungsmessung am oberen Sprunggelenk unter Serrapeptase—eine prospektive Studie." ["Reduction of Postoperative Swelling. Objective Measurement of Swelling of the Upper Ankle Joint in Treatment with Serrapeptase—A Prospective Study."] *MMW Fortschritte der Medizin* 107, no. 4 (1989): 67–8, 71-2. PMID:2647603.

27. Guerra, Carlos, et al. "Glutathione and Adaptive Immune Responses Against Mycobacterium Tuberculosis Infection in Healthy and HIV-Infected Individuals." *PLOS One* 6, no. 12 (2011): e28378. doi:10.1371/journal.pone.0028378.

28. Yatmaz, Selcuk, et al. "Glutathione Peroxidase-1 Reduces Influenza A Virus–Induced Lung Inflammation." *American Journal of Respiratory Cell and Molecular Biology* 48, no. 1 (2013): 17–26. doi:10.1165/rcmb.2011-0345OC.

29. Ghezzi, Pietro. "Role of Glutathione in Immunity and Inflammation in the Lung." *International Journal of General Medicine* 4 (2011): 105–13. doi:10.2147/IJGM.S15618.

30. Pedersen, Bente Klarlund. "Anti-Inflammatory Effects of Exercise: Role in Diabetes and Cardiovascular Disease." *European Journal of Clinical Investigation* 47, no. 8 (2017): 600–611. doi:10.1111/eci.12781.

31. Khazaei, Majid. "Chronic Low-Grade Inflammation after Exercise: Controversies." *Iranian Journal of Basic Medical Sciences* 15, no. 5 (2012): 1008–9. PMID:23495361.

32. Pedersen, Bente Klarlund. "Anti-Inflammatory Effects of Exercise: Role in Diabetes and Cardiovascular Disease." *European Journal of Clinical Investigation* 47, no. 8 (2017): 600–611. doi:10.1111/eci.12781.

33. Khazaei, Majid. "Chronic Low-Grade Inflammation after Exercise: Controversies." *Iranian Journal of Basic Medical Sciences* 15, no. 5 (2012): 1008–9. PMID:23495361.

34. Shete, Sanjay Uddhav, et al. "Effect of Yoga Training on Inflammatory Cytokines and C-Reactive Protein in Employees of Small-Scale Industries." *Journal of Education and Health Promotion* 6 (2017): 76. doi:10.4103/jehp.jehp_65_17.

35. Kiecolt-Glaser, Janice K., et al. "Stress, Inflammation, and Yoga Practice." *Psychosomatic Medicine* 72, no. 2 (2010): 113–21. doi:10.1097/PSY.0b013-e3181cb9377.

36. Avci, Pinar, et al. "Low-Level Laser (Light) Therapy (LLLT) in Skin: Stimulating, Healing, Restoring." *Seminars in Cutaneous Medicine and Surgery* 32, no. 1 (2013): 41–52. PMID:24049929.

37. Hamblin, Michael R. "Mechanisms and Applications of the Anti-inflammatory Effects of Photobiomodulation." *AIMS Biophysics* 4, no. 3 (2017): 337–361. doi:10.3934/biophy.2017.3.337.

Chapter 10: Enhance Your Sleep

1. Poe, Gina R. "Sleep Is for Forgetting." *Journal of Neuroscience* 37, no. 3 (2017): 464–473. doi:10.1523/JNEUROSCI.0820-16.2017; Cousins, James N., et al. "Chapter 2: The Impact of Sleep Deprivation on Declarative Memory." *Progress in Brain Research* 246 (2019): 27–53. doi:10.1016/bs.pbr.2019.01.007; Reddy, Oliver Cameron and Ysbrand D. van der Werf. "The Sleeping Brain: Harnessing the Power of the Glymphatic System through Lifestyle Choices." *Brain Sciences* 10, no. 11 (2020): 868. doi:10.3390/brainsci10110868.

2. Taheri, Shahrad, et al. "Short Sleep Duration Is Associated with Reduced Leptin, Elevated Ghrelin, and Increased Body Mass Index." *PLOS Medicine* 1, no. 3 (2004): e62. doi:10.1371/journal.pmed.0010062.

3. Hanlon, Erin C., et al. "Sleep Restriction Enhances the Daily Rhythm of Circulating Levels of Endocannabinoid 2-Arachidonoylglycerol." *Sleep* 39, no. 3 (2016): 653–64. doi:10.5665/sleep.5546.

4. St-Onge, Marie-Pierre, et al. "Sleep Restriction Leads to Increased Activation of Brain Regions Sensitive to Food Stimuli." *The American Journal of Clinical Nutrition* 95, no. 4 (2012): 818–24. doi:10.3945/ajcn.111.027383.

5. Ali, Tauseef, et al. "Sleep, Immunity and Inflammation in Gastrointestinal Disorders." *World Journal of Gastroenterology* 19, no. 48 (2013): 9231–9. doi:10.3748/wjg.v19.i48.9231.

6. Irwin, Michael R., et al. "Sleep Loss Activates Cellular Inflammatory Signaling." *Biological Psychiatry* 64, no. 6 (2008): 538–40. doi:10.1016/j.biopsych.2008.05.004.

7. Gamaldo, Charlene E., et al. "The Sleep-Immunity Relationship." *Neurologic Clinics* 30, no. 4 (2012): 1313–43. doi:10.1016/j.ncl.2012.08.007.

8. Chang, Hung-Ming, et al. "Sleep Deprivation Predisposes Liver to Oxidative Stress and Phospholipid Damage: A Quantitative Molecular Imaging Study." *Journal of Anatomy* 212, no. 3 (2008): 295–305. doi:10.1111/j.1469-7580.2008.00860.x.

9. Buxton, Orfeu M., et al. "Sleep Restriction for One Week Reduces Insulin Sensitivity in Healthy Men." *Diabetes* 59, no. 9 (2010): 2126–33. doi:10.2337/db09-0699.

10. Hirshkowitz, Max, et al. "National Sleep Foundation's Sleep Time Duration Recommendations: Methodology and Results Summary." *Sleep Health* 1, no. 1 (2015): 40–43. doi:10.1016/j.sleh.2014.12.010; Lichtenstein, Gary R. "The Importance of Sleep." *Gastroenterology & Hepatology* 11, no. 12 (2015): 790.

11. Chaput, Jean-Philippe, et al. "Sleeping Hours: What Is the Ideal Number and How Does Age Impact This?" *Nature and Science of Sleep* 10 (2018): 421–430. doi:10.2147/NSS.S163071.

12. Ohayon, Maurice, et al. "National Sleep Foundation's Sleep Quality Recommendations: First Report." *Sleep Health: Journal of the National Sleep Foundation* 3, no. 1 (2017): 6–19. doi:10.1016/j.sleh.2016.11.006.

13. Massa, Jennifer, et al. "Vitamin D and Actigraphic Sleep Outcomes in Older Community-Dwelling Men: The MrOS Sleep Study." *Sleep* 38, no. 2 (2015): 251–7. doi:10.5665/sleep.4408.

14. Li, X., et al. "The Association Between Serum Vitamin D and Obstructive Sleep Apnea: An Updated Meta-Analysis." *Respiratory Research* 21, no. 294 (2020). doi:10.1186/s12931-020-01554-2.

15. Huang, Wenyu, et al. "Circadian Rhythms, Sleep, and Metabolism." *The Journal of Clinical Investigation* 121, no. 6 (2011): 2133–41. doi:10.1172/JCI46043.

16. Zisapel, Nava. "New Perspectives on the Role of Melatonin in Human Sleep, Circadian Rhythms, and Their Regulation." *British Journal of Pharmacology* 175, no. 16 (2018): 3190–3199. doi:10.1111/bph.14116.

17. Jamshed, Humaira, et al. "Early Time-Restricted Feeding Improves 24-Hour Glucose Levels and Affects Markers of the Circadian Clock, Aging, and Autophagy in Humans." *Nutrients* 11, no. 6 (2019): 1234. doi:10.3390/nu11061234.

18. Pejovic, Slobodanka, et al. "Effects of Recovery Sleep After One Work Week of Mild Sleep Restriction on Interleukin 6 and Cortisol Secretion and Daytime Sleepiness and Performance." *American Journal of Physiology, Endocrinology, and Metabolism* 305, no. 7 (2013): E890–6. doi:10.1152/ajpendo.00301.2013.

19. Madjd, A., et al. "Effects of Consuming Later Evening Meal vs. Earlier Evening Meal on Weight Loss During a Weight Loss Diet: A Randomised Clinical Trial." *British Journal of Nutrition* 126, no. 4 (2021): 632–640. doi:10.1017/S0007114520004456.

20. Wurtman, Richard J. and Judith J. Wurtman. "Do Carbohydrates Affect Food Intake via Neurotransmitter Activity?" *Appetite* 11, no. 1 (1988): 42–47. doi:10.1016/S0195-6663(88)80045-X.

21. Ebrahim, Irshaad O., et al. "Alcohol and Sleep I: Effects on Normal Sleep." *Alcoholism, Clinical and Experimental Research* 37, no. 4 (2013): 539–49. doi:10.1111/acer.12006; Brower, K.J. "Alcohol's Effects on Sleep in Alcoholics." *Alcohol Research & Health* 25, no. 2 (2001): 110–25.

22. Stutz, Jan, et al. "Effects of Evening Exercise on Sleep in Healthy Participants: A Systematic Review and Meta-Analysis." *Sports Medicine* (Auckland, NZ) 49, no. 2 (2019): 269–287. doi:10.1007/s40279-018-1015-0.

23. Burkhart, Kimberly and James R. Phelps. "Amber Lenses to Block Blue Light and Improve Sleep: A Randomized Trial." *Chronobiology International* 26, no. 8 (2009): 1602–12. doi:10.3109/07420520903523719.

24. Pacheco, Danielle. "The Best Temperature for Sleep." The Sleep Foundation. SleepFoundation.org /bedroom-environment/best-temperature-for-sleep.

25. Karacan, I., et al. "Effects of High Ambient Temperature on Sleep in Young Men." *Aviation, Space, and Environmental Medicine* 49, no. 7 (1978): 855–60.

26. Masters, Alina, et al. "Melatonin, the Hormone of Darkness: From Sleep Promotion to Ebola Treatment." *Brain Disorders & Therapy* 4, no. 1 (2014): 1000151. doi:10.4172/2168-975X.1000151; Vriend, Jerry and Russel J. Reiter. "Melatonin Feedback on Clock Genes: A Theory Involving the Proteasome." *Journal of Pineal Research* 58, no. 1 (2015): 1–11. doi:10.1111/jpi.12189.

27. Arendt, Josephine and Debra Jean Skene. "Melatonin as a Chronobiotic." *Sleep Medicine Reviews* 9, no. 1 (2005): 25–39. doi:10.1016/j. smrv.2004.05.002; Brzezinski, Amnon, et al. "Effects of Exogenous Melatonin on Sleep: A Meta-Analysis." *Sleep Medicine* Reviews 9, no. 1 (2005): 41–50. doi:10.1016/j.smrv.2004.06.004.

28. Wienecke, Elmar and Claudia Nolden. "Langzeit-HRV-Analyse zeigt Stressreduktion durch Magnesiumzufuhr." ["Long-Term HRV Analysis Shows Stress Reduction by Magnesium Intake."] *MMW Fortschritte der Medizin* 158, no. 6 (2016): 12–16. doi:10.1007/s15006-016-9054-7.

29. Poleszak, Ewa. "Benzodiazepine/GABA(A) Receptors Are Involved in Magnesium-Induced Anxiolytic-Like Behavior in Mice." *Pharmacological Reports: PR* 60, no. 4 (2008): 483–9. PMID:18799816; Uygun, David S., et al. "Bottom-Up versus Top-Down Induction of Sleep by Zolpidem Acting on Histaminergic and Neocortex Neurons." *The Journal of Neuroscience* 36, no. 44 (2016): 11171–11184. doi:10.1523/JNEUROSCI.3714-15.2016.

30. Durlach, Jean, et al. "Biorhythms and Possible Central Regulation of Magnesium Status, Phototherapy, Darkness Therapy, and Chronopathological Forms of Magnesium Depletion." *Magnesium Research* 15, nos. 1–2 (2002): 49–66. PMID:12030424.

31. Nobre, A., et al. "L-Theanine, a Natural Constituent in Tea, and Its Effect on Mental State." *Asia Pacific Journal of Clinical Nutrition* 17, no. 1 (2008): 167–168. PMID:18296328; Abdou, A., et al. "Relaxation and Immunity Enhancement Effects of Gamma-Aminobutyric Acid (GABA) Administration in Humans." *Biofactors* 26, no. 3 (2006): 201–208. doi:10.1002/biof.5520260305.

32. Hidese, S., et al. "Effects of L-Theanine Administration on Stress-Related Symptoms and Cognitive Functions in Healthy Adults: A Randomized Controlled Trial." *Nutrients* 11, no. 10 (2019): 2362. doi:10.3390 /nu11102362.

33. Bannai, Makoto and Nobuhiro Kawai. "New Therapeutic Strategy for Amino Acid Medicine: Glycine Improves the Quality of Sleep." *Journal of Pharmacological Sciences* 118, no. 2 (2012): 145–8. doi:10.1254 /jphs.11r04fm.

34. Zhao, Jiexiu, et al. "Red Light and the Sleep Quality and Endurance Performance of Chinese Female Basketball Players." *Journal of Athletic Training* 47, no. 6 (2012): 673–8. doi:10.4085/1062-6050-47.6.08.

35. Reyner, L.A. and J.A. Horne. "Suppression of Sleepiness in Drivers: Combination of Caffeine with a Short Nap." *Psychophysiology* 34, no. 6 (1997): 721–5. doi:10.1111/j.1469-8986.1997.tb02148.x.

Chapter 11: Additional Strategies for Women

1. Heldring, Nina, et al. "Estrogen Receptors: How Do They Signal and What Are Their Targets." *Physiological Reviews* 87, no. 3 (2007): 905–31. doi:10.1152/physrev .00026.2006.

2. Andrabi, Syed Suhail, et al. "Neurosteroids and Ischemic Stroke: Progesterone a Promising Agent in Reducing the Brain Injury in Ischemic Stroke." *Journal of Environmental Pathology, Toxicology, and Oncology* 36, no. 3 (2017): 191–205. doi:10.1615 /JEnvironPatholToxicolOncol.20170; van Wingen, G., et al. "Progesterone Selectively Increases Amygdala Reactivity in Women." *Molecular Psychiatry* 13 (2008): 325–333. doi:10.1038/sj.mp.4002030.

3. Santoro, N., et al. "Factors Related to Declining Luteal Function in Women During the Menopausal Transition." *The Journal of Clinical Endocrinology & Metabolism* 93, no. 5 (2008): 1711–21. doi:10.1210/jc.2007-2165.

4. Cavalieri, Ercole L. and Eleanor G. Rogan. "Depurinating Estrogen-DNA Adducts, Generators of Cancer Initiation: Their Minimization Leads to Cancer Prevention." *Clinical and Translational Medicine* 5, no. 1 (2016): 12. doi:10.1186/s40169-016-0088-3; Samavat, Hamed and Mindy S. Kurzer. "Estrogen Metabolism and Breast Cancer." *Cancer Letters* 356, no. 2 Pt A (2015): 231–43. doi:10.1016/j.canlet.2014.04.018.

5. Plottel, Claudia S. and Martin J. Blaser. "Microbiome and Malignancy." *Cell Host & Microbe* 10, no. 4 (2011): 324–35. doi:10.1016/j.chom.2011.10.003.

6. Flores, R., et al. "Fecal Microbial Determinants of Fecal and Systemic Estrogens and Estrogen Metabolites: A Cross-Sectional Study." *Journal of Translational Medicine* 10, no. 253 (2012). doi:10.1186/1479-5876-10-253.

7. Thomson, Cynthia A., et al. "Chemopreventive Properties of 3,3'-diindolylmethane in Breast Cancer: Evidence from Experimental and Human Studies." *Nutrition Reviews* 74, no. 7 (2016): 432–43. doi:10.1093/nutrit/nuw010; Rajoria, Shilpi, et al. "3,3'-diindolylmethane Modulates Estrogen Metabolism in Patients with Thyroid Proliferative Disease: A Pilot Study." *Thyroid* 21, no. 3 (2011): 299–304. doi:10.1089/thy.2010.0245.

8. Thomson, Cynthia A., et al. "Chemopreventive Properties of 3,3'-diindolylmethane in Breast Cancer: Evidence from Experimental and Human Studies." *Nutrition Reviews* 74, no. 7 (2016): 432–43. doi:10.1093/nutrit/nuw010; De Santi, Mauro, et al. "Inhibition of Testosterone Aromatization by the Indole-3-carbinol Derivative CTet in CYP19A1-overexpressing MCF-7 Breast Cancer Cells." *Anti-Cancer Agents in Medicinal Chemistry* 15, no. 7 (2015): 896–904. doi:10.2174/1871520615666150121123053.

9. Tortorella, Stephanie M., et al. "Dietary Sulforaphane in Cancer Chemoprevention: The Role of Epigenetic Regulation and HDAC Inhibition." *Antioxidants & Redox Signaling* 22, no. 16 (2015): 1382–424. doi:10.1089/ars.2014.6097; Su, Xuling, et al. "Anticancer Activity of Sulforaphane: The Epigenetic Mechanisms and the Nrf2 Signaling Pathway." *Oxidative Medicine and Cellular Longevity* 2018 (2018): 5438179. doi:10.1155/2018/5438179.

10. United States Department of Agriculture. *Dietary Guidelines for Americans 2020–2025.* DietaryGuidelines.gov. DietaryGuidelines.gov/sites/default/files/2021-03/Dietary_Guidelines_for_Americans-2020-2025.pdf.

11. Kurzer, M.S. and X. Xu. "Dietary Phytoestrogens." *The Annual Review of Nutrition* 17 (1997): 353–81. doi:10.1146/annurev.nutr.17.1.353.

12. Tham, Doris M., et al. "Potential Health Benefits of Dietary Phytoestrogens: A Review of the Clinical, Epidemiological, and Mechanistic Evidence." *The Journal of Clinical Endocrinology & Metabolism* 83, no. 7 (1998): 2223–2235. doi:10.1210/jcem.83.7.4752.

13. Hwang, Chang Sun, et al. "Isoflavone Metabolites and Their In Vitro Dual Functions: They Can Act as an Estrogenic Agonist or Antagonist Depending on the Estrogen Concentration." *The Journal of Steroid Biochemistry and Molecular Biology* 101, nos. 4–5 (2006): 246–53. doi:10.1016/j.jsbmb.2006.06.020.

14. Phipps, W.R., et al. "Effect of Flaxseed Ingestion on the Menstrual Cycle." *The Journal of Clinical Endocrinology & Metabolism* 77, no. 5 (1993): 1215–9. doi:10.1210/jcem.77.5.8077314; Ivonee, M.C., et al. "The Potential Health Effects of Dietary Phytoestrogens." *British Journal of Pharmacology* 174, no. 11 (2017): 1263–1280. doi:10.1111/bph.13622; Bryant, M., et al. "Effect of Consumption of Soy Isoflavones on Behavioural, Somatic, and Affective Symptoms in Women with Premenstrual Syndrome." *British Journal of Nutrition* 93, no. 5 (2005): 731–9. doi:10.1079/bjn20041396.

15. American Thyroid Association. General Information/Press Room. Thyroid.org/media-main/press-room/.

16. American Thyroid Association. General Information/Press Room. Thyroid.org/media-main/press-room/.

17. Koutras, D.A. "Disturbances of Menstruation in Thyroid Disease." *Annals of the New York Academy of Sciences* 816 (1997): 280–4. doi:10.1111/j.1749-6632.1997.tb52152.x.

18. Santin, Ana Paula and Tania Weber Furlanetto. "Role of Estrogen in Thyroid Function and Growth Regulation." *Journal of Thyroid Research* 2011 (2011): 875125. doi:10.4061/2011/875125.

19. Santin, Ana Paula and Tania Weber Furlanetto. "Role of Estrogen in Thyroid Function and Growth Regulation."*Journal of Thyroid Research* 2011 (2011): 875125. doi:10.4061/2011/875125.

20. Walter, Kimberly N., et al. "Elevated Thyroid Stimulating Hormone Is Associated with Elevated Cortisol in Healthy Young Men and Women." *Thyroid Research* 5, no. 1 (2012): 13. doi:10.1186/1756-6614-5-13; Helmreich, Dana L., et al. "Relation Between the Hypothalamic-Pituitary-Thyroid (HPT) Axis and the Hypothalamic-Pituitary-Adrenal (HPA) Axis During Repeated Stress." *Neuroendocrinology* 81, no. 3 (2005): 183–92. doi:10.1159/000087001.

21. Vojdani, Aristo, et al. "Environmental Triggers and Autoimmunity." *Autoimmune Diseases* 2014 (2014): 798029. doi:10.1155/2014/798029.

22. Kumarathilaka, Prasanna, et al. "Perchlorate as an Emerging Contaminant in Soil, Water, and Food." *Chemosphere* 150 (2016): 667–677. doi:10.1016/j.chemosphere.2016.01.109.

23. Blount, Benjamin C., et al. "Urinary Perchlorate and Thyroid Hormone Levels in Adolescent and Adult Men and Women Living in the United States." *Environmental Health Perspectives* 114, no. 12 (2006): 1865–71. doi:10.1289/ehp.9466; Leung, Angela M., et al. "Perchlorate, Iodine, and the Thyroid." *Best Practice & Research: Clinical Endocrinology & Metabolism* 24, no. 1 (2010): 133–41. doi:10.1016/j.beem.2009.08.009.

24. Wolff, J. "Perchlorate and the Thyroid Gland." *Pharmacological Reviews* 50, no. 1 (1998): 89–105. PMID:9549759; Turyk, Mary E., et al. "Relationships of Thyroid Hormones with Polychlorinated Biphenyls, Dioxins, Furans, and DDE in Adults." *Environmental Health Perspectives* 115, no. 8 (2007): 1197–203. doi:10.1289/ehp.10179.

25. Turyk, Mary E., et al. "Relationships of Thyroid Hormones with Polychlorinated Biphenyls, Dioxins, Furans, and DDE in Adults." *Environmental Health Perspectives* 115, no. 8 (2007): 1197–203. doi:10.1289/ehp.10179.

26. Zoeller, R. Thomas. "Environmental Chemicals as Thyroid Hormone Analogues: New Studies Indicate that Thyroid Hormone Receptors are Targets of Industrial Chemicals?" *Molecular and Cellular Endocrinology* 242 (2005): 10–15. doi:10.1016/j.mce.2005.07.006.

27. Li, Na, et al. "Dibutyl Phthalate Contributes to the Thyroid Receptor Antagonistic Activity in Drinking Water Processes." *Environmental Science & Technology* 44, no. 17 (2010): 6863–8. doi:10.1021/es101254c.

28. Hinther, Ashley, et al. "Effects of Triclocarban, Triclosan, and Methyl Triclosan on Thyroid Hormone Action and Stress in Frog and Mammalian Culture Systems." *Environmental Science & Technology* 45, no. 12 (2011): 5395–402. doi:10.1021/es1041942; Louis, Gwendolyn W., et al. "Effects of Chronic Exposure to Triclosan on Reproductive and Thyroid Endpoints in the Adult Wistar Female Rat." *Journal of Toxicology and Environmental Health* 80, no. 4 (2017): 236–249. doi:10.1080/15287394.2017.1287029.

29. Rice, Kevin M., et al. "Environmental Mercury and Its Toxic Effects." *Journal of Preventive Medicine and Public Health = Yebang Uihakhoe chi* 47, no. 2 (2014): 74–83. doi:10.3961/jpmph.2014.47.2.74.

30. Orihuela, Daniel. "Aluminium Effects on Thyroid Gland Function: Iodide Uptake, Hormone Biosynthesis, and Secretion." *Journal of Inorganic Biochemistry* 105, no. 11 (2011): 1464–8. doi:10.1016/j.jinorgbio.2011.08.004; Watad, Abdulla, et al. "Autoimmune/Inflammatory Syndrome Induced by Adjuvants and Thyroid Autoimmunity." *Frontiers in Endocrinology* 7 (2017): 150. doi:10.3389/fendo.2016.00150.

31. Duan, Lihua, et al. "Regulation of Inflammation in Autoimmune Disease." *Journal of Immunology Research* 2019 (2019): 7403796. doi:10.1155/2019/7403796.

32. Severo, Juliana Soares, et al. "The Role of Zinc in Thyroid Hormones Metabolism." *International Journal for Vitamin and Nutrition Research. Internationale Zeitschrift fur Vitamin- und Ernahrungsforschung. Journal international de vitaminologie et de nutrition* 89, nos. 1–2 (2019): 80–88. doi:10.1024/0300-9831/a000262.

33. Arthur, J.R., et al. "The Role of Selenium in Thyroid Hormone Metabolism and Effects of Selenium Deficiency on Thyroid Hormone and Iodine Metabolism." *Biological Trace Element Research* 34, no. 3 (1992): 321–5. doi:10.1007/BF02783686; Ventura, Mara, et al. "Selenium and Thyroid Disease: From Pathophysiology to Treatment." *International Journal of Endocrinology* 2017 (2017): 1297658. doi:10.1155/2017/1297658.

34. Felker, Peter, et al. "Concentrations of Thiocyanate and Goitrin in Human Plasma, Their Precursor Concentrations in Brassica Vegetables, and Associated Potential Risk for Hypothyroidism." *Nutrition Reviews* 74, no. 4 (2016): 248–258. doi:10.1093/nutrit/nuv110.

35. Calsolaro, Valeria, et al. "Thyroid Disrupting Chemicals." *International Journal of Molecular Sciences* 18, no. 12 (2017): 2583. doi:10.3390/ijms18122583.

Chapter 12: Maintain Motivation

1. America Psychological Association. "Multitasking: Switching Costs." American Psychological Association. APA.org/research/action/multitask.

2. Schultz, W. "Dopamine Signals for Reward Value and Risk: Basic and Recent Data." *Behavioral and Brain Functions* 6, no. 24 (2010). doi:10.1186/1744-9081-6-24.

3. Ranganathan, Vinoth K., et al. "From Mental Power to Muscle Power—Gaining Strength by Using the Mind." *Neuropsychologia* 42, no. 7 (2004): 944–56. doi:10.1016/j.neuropsychologia.2003.11.018; Cisek, P. and J. Kalaska. "Neural Correlates of Mental Rehearsal in Dorsal Premotor Cortex." *Nature* 431 (2004): 993–996. doi:10.1038/nature03005; Natraj, Nikhilesh and Karunesh Ganguly. "Shaping Reality Through Mental Rehearsal." *Neuron* 97, no. 5 (2018): 998–1000. doi:10.1016/j.neuron.2018.02.017; Roure, R., et al. "Autonomic Nervous System Responses Correlate with Mental Rehearsal in Volleyball Training." *European Journal of Applied Physiology* 78 (1998): 99–108. doi:10.1007/s004210050393.

4. Ranganathan, Vinoth K., et al. "From Mental Power to Muscle Power—Gaining Strength by Using the Mind." *Neuropsychologia* 42, no. 7 (2004): 944–56. doi:10.1016/j.neuropsychologia.2003.11.018.

5. Liu, Z., et al. "Learning Motivational Significance of Visual Cues for Reward Schedules Requires Rhinal Cortex." *Nature Neuroscience* 3, no. 12 (2000): 1307–15. doi:10.1038/81841.

6. Harkin, Benjamin, et al. "Does Monitoring Goal Progress Promote Goal Attainment? A Meta-Analysis of the Experimental Evidence." *Psychological Bulletin* 142, no. 2 (2016): 198–229. doi:10.1037/bul0000025.

7. Amabile, Teresa M. and Steven J. Kramer. "The Power of Small Wins." *Harvard Business Review* 89, no. 5 (May 2011).

8. Phillips, Allison L. and Benjamin Gardner. "Habitual Exercise Instigation (vs. Execution) Predicts Healthy Adults' Exercise Frequency." *Health Psychology* 35, no. 1 (2016): 69–77. doi:10.1037/hea0000249.

9. Byrne, N., et al. "Intermittent Energy Restriction Improves Weight Loss Efficiency in Obese Men: The MATADOR Study." *International Journal of Obesity* 42 (2018): 129–138. doi:10.1038/ijo.2017.206.

Chapter 14: Do What's Best for You

1. Crowley, Jennifer, et al. "Nutrition in Medical Education: A Systematic Review." *The Lancet. Planetary Health* 3, no. 9 (2019): e379–e389. doi:10.1016/S2542-5196(19)30171-8.

2. Manninen, Anssi H. "Very-Low-Carbohydrate Diets and Preservation of Muscle Mass." *Nutrition & Metabolism* 3, no. 9. (2006). doi:10.1186/1743-7075-3-9.

3. van den Beld, Annewieke W., et al. "The Physiology of Endocrine Systems with Aging." *The Lancet. Diabetes & Endocrinology* 6, no. 8 (2018): 647–658. doi:10.1016/S2213-8587(18)30026-3.

4. Xu, C., et al. "Aging Progression of Human Gut Microbiota." *BMC Microbiology* 19, no. 236 (2019). doi:10.1186/s12866-019-1616-2.

Index

capsule form, avoiding during a fast, 74
during a fast, 71, 80
improve effectiveness of a fast, 149–150
making your own pre-workout supplement, 74
recommended, 123–127
reducing inflammation, 162
for sleep, 177–178
tips for choosing a high-quality, 123
turmeric, 156
Sweeteners, 69, 70, 73, 80, 119, 120
Synaptic plasticity, 57, 59

T

Tea, 66, 69. *See also* Green tea
Teff, 90–91, 120
"The Four Pillars," 196–197
Thirty-six hour fast, 144, 146
Thyroid health
getting tested for thyroid issues, 191
gluten and, 92
seaweed and, 94, 98
thyroid issues in women, 27, 188–192
Thyroid-stimulating hormone (TSH), 189
Thyroxine (T4), 189
Tobacco/smoking, 75
Toothpaste, 74
Toxins, 159–160, 186, 187, 190, 192
Transcription factor EB (TFEB), 72
Triclosan, 160, 190
Triglycerides, 15, 18, 47
Triiodothyronine (T3), 189
Turkey/turkey sticks/jerky, 90, 99, 102
Turmeric, 66, 71, 72, 147, 148, 156
Twelve-hour fasting window/twelve-hour fast, 30, 32, 33, 133
Twenty-four-hour alternate-day fast, 26, 136
2MAD (two meals a day), 114
Type 2 diabetes, 43
Tyrosine, 94, 98, 149–150

U

Undereating, 128
Unsaturated fats. *See* Monounsaturated fats; Polyunsaturated fats

V

Vaping, 75
Varicella-zoster virus (VZV), 161
Vascular endothelial growth factor (VEGF), 31, 39
Vegan/vegetarian diet
about, 112–113, 115
B$_{12}$ deficiency and, 125
breaking a fast meals, 101
fats and, 67
lean protein in mini break-fast meal for, 90–91
omega-3 fatty acids and, 124
vitamin D deficiency, 126
Vegetable oils, 95, 120
Vegetables
breaking a fast and, 92
cruciferous, 95, 99–100, 187, 192
in normal-size meal when breaking a fast, 95
in pre-fast meal, 67
Venison jerky/sticks, 99
Very low-density lipoprotein (VLDL), 47
Visceral fat, 39, 85
Visualization, 202–203
Vitamin B$_{12}$, 113
Vitamin B complex, 125
Vitamin C, 71, 80, 98, 125, 127
Vitamin D, 125–126, 127, 170
Vitamin deficiency, 130

W

Water intake. *See* Hydration
Weight gain, sleep and, 168
Weight loss, 138
author's personal story about, 7–8
intermittent fasting causing, 38–39
negativity from others and, 219–220
pace of, 217
Whey protein powder, 91
White blood cells, 44, 48, 149, 162
White fat, 31, 39, 50
Whole-day fasting, 144
Wild Alaskan salmon, 118
Wild rice, 120
Women
caffeine intake, 75
dairy intake and, 126
estrogen dominance and, 183–187
intermittent fasting for, 26–27

seaweed for, 94
shellfish for, when breaking a fast, 96
thyroid issues, 188–192
Workout(s)/working out. *See also* Exercise
adding an upper/lower split, 148–149
benefits, 77
breaking a fast and, 103–104
creating a habit for, 204
drinking beet juice before a, 155
in a fasted state, 145
during fasting window, 77–78
making your own pre-workout supplement, 74
micro goals for, 202
preferred schedule for, 33
at varying times of the day, 143

X

Xenoestrogens, 186, 187
Xylitol, 73, 74

Y

Yerba mate, 83
Yoga, 79, 164, 175
Yogurt, 96, 99, 100, 101

Z

Zinc, 192